# THE OCULAR FUNDUS

A Color Atlas

by

HANS-WALTHER LARSEN, M.D.
Professor of Ophthalmology,
University of Copenhagen,
School of Medicine,
Department of Ophthalmology,
Gentofte Hospital.

523 color photographs
illustrating common and rare fundus diseases
and a descriptive text including considerations
of differential diagnosis

W. B. SAUNDERS COMPANY
Philadelphia · London · Toronto

THE OCULAR FUNDUS has been designed by the author and the publisher, Munksgaard, in collaboration with the printers C. Hamburger, Copenhagen. The type-face used is French Antiqua. The book is printed on coated paper from Papierfabrik Scheufelen. Photographic processing by Brdr. Jacobsen. Blocks by Rotogravure A/S. Cover design by Ib K. Olsen. Bound by Durland & Co. Offset printing of the text by Villadsen & Christensen, Copenhagen.

Originally published by Munksgaard, Copenhagen

© Munksgaard, Copenhagen, Denmark 1976

ISBN 87-16-02149-5

Published simultaneously in the USA by
W. B. Saunders Company

L.C.C.N. 75-31301

ISBN 0-7216-5631-5

# Preface

The present Atlas, which is a revised and condensed edition of my "Manual and Color Atlas of the Ocular Fundus" should fullfill the need for a detailed but rather inexpensive color atlas of the ocular fundus.

The Atlas is intended especially for ophthalmologists and residents in ophthalmology, but should also give other clinicians—internists, neurologists, neurosurgeons, doctors in general practice, medical students, etc., who wish to perform an ophthalmoscopy themselves or interpret the observations of the ophthalmologist—the possibility of studying these changes by means of fundus photographs in color.

For technical reasons the description of the various fundus diseases is placed on left-hand pages as close as possible to the illustrations. The picture and a short descriptive text are placed on right-hand pages.

All photographs were taken by the author with a Zeiss Fundus Camera or a Nikon Hand Fundus Camera on Agfacolor Reversal Film CT 18 or Kodachrome II Daylight Film K 135. The pictures are reproduced from color copies as near as possible to the original diapositives. The montage photographs are enlarged 1.75 times and the other photographs 2.5 times.

In addition to the ordinary objectives with which 30° of the fundus can be photographed, a special objective was used in connection with the Zeiss Fundus Camera, permitting only 15° of the fundus to be photographed. In the text, the term "15°" refers to pictures taken with this special objective.

The pictures are a selection of fundus photographs from in-patients and out-patients at the Steno Memorial Hospital (Niels Steensens Hospital, Gentofte, Denmark), the Eye Clinics and Eye Departments at the Copenhagen University Hospitals (Rigshospitalet, Kommunehospitalet and Gentofte Hospital) and my own private practice, during the period 1957—1968.

I am very grateful to all my colleagues who referred their patients to the above mentioned clinics for further study and fundus photography and to all those patients who made this extensive study possible.

Finally, I would like to express my deep indebtedness to Messrs. Munksgaard for giving me the opportunity to publish this Atlas in its present form.

Hans-Walther Larsen

# CONTENTS

# The Normal Fundus
### (Figures 1—11)

The appearance of the normal fundus varies within wide limits.

The optic disc is the most obvious feature in the ophthalmoscopic view of the fundus. It measures about 1.5 mm in diameter and corresponds in position with the entrance of the optic nerve into the bulb. It is seen as a pale, round or oval, well-defined structure, with a pink or yellowish-red tint, which contrasts notably with the color of the fundus.

The central retinal artery and vein normally appear close to each other at the nasal side of the center of the optic disc. Within the disc margin, they usually divide into a large superior and inferior branch and soon after into temporal and nasal branches. The four principal divisions supply the four quadrants of the fundus and take a slightly sinuous course as they proceed into their respective quadrants, dividing dichotomously into innumerable branches (Fig. 1). In addition to these main divisions, one or more small nasal arteries are often seen to run from the nasal side of the optic disc into the retina, and one or two small macular arteries may run temporally towards the macula (Figs. 1 and 3). In the macular area, there is a capillary-free zone of about 0.5 mm corresponding to the fovea centralis (Figs. 1—2 and 4—8).

The arteries appear lighter red and narrower than the dark-red or purplish veins, and normally the arteriovenous ratio is about 2:3. The retinal vessels have a continuous yellow-white axial light reflex, and the arterial reflex is more brilliant than the venous reflex (Fig. 1).

The macula is situated about two disc diameters temporal to and slightly below the optic disc (Figs. 1—2 and 4—8). It is a horizontally oval area about the same size as the disc, appearing slightly deeper red or darker in color than the adjacent fundus and surrounded by an annular light reflex (Figs. 2, 4, 5, 7). At the center of the macula, there is a small depression, the fovea, indicated by a deep-red or red-brown color and a small brilliant reflex, the foveal reflex (Fig. 2).

As the light from the ophthalmoscope is moved, shimmering reflexes frequently become apparent. The fundus reflexes

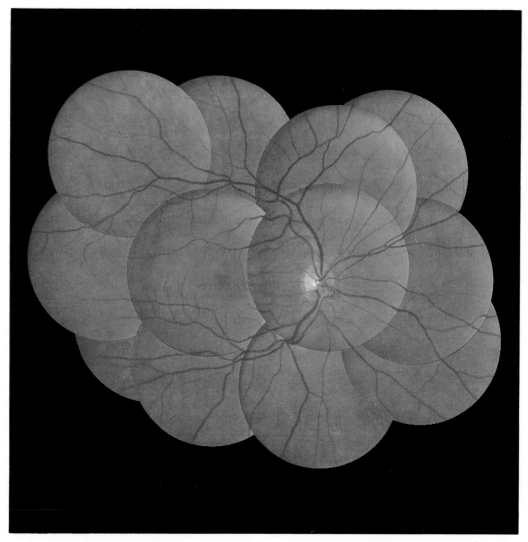

*Figure 1. Composite picture. Right eye. Normal appearance of a medium pigmented fundus. The fundus has a uniform, warm red color. The optic disc and the retinal vessels are normal.*

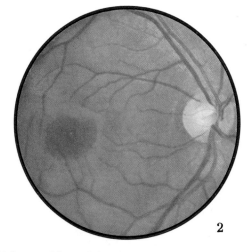

2

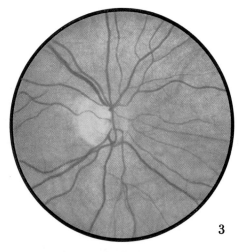

3

*Right eye. Normal fundus in a young person.*

*Right eye. Normal appearance of a lightly pigmented fundus.*

are most prominent in children and young individuals (Figs. 2 and 7) and show a gradual decrease as age advances (Fig. 6).

The color of the fundus varies considerably, depending on the amount and distribution of pigment in the individual retina and choroid.

In lightly pigmented subjects the fundus assumes an orange-red color and sometimes the choroidal vessels are seen plainly (Fig. 3). In medium pigmented subjects the color is more red (Figs. 1—2), while in heavily pigmented subjects it is dark-red (Figs. 8—9), red-brown (Fig. 4) or even brownish-green (Figs. 5—7). If the choroidal pigmentation is heavier than the retinal pigmentation, it may give rise to the appearance of a tessellated or tigroid fundus (Figs. 8—9).

In very lightly pigmented subjects with extensive exposure of the choroidal vessels (Fig. 11), the ophthalmoscopic appearance may resemble that in albinism, but in the former condition, pseudo-albinism, the macula and fovea remain normal (Fig. 10) in contrast to true albinism (Fig. 12).

The retinal and partly also the choroidal blood circulation can be visualized by fluorescein angiography.

After injection of a solution of sodium fluorescein into the cubital vein, the dye normally appears in the retinal arteries after 10 to 15 seconds. The arterial phase is followed by arteriovenous and venous phases. Normally the retinal vessels show no leakage of dye, and fluorescein has left the retinal circulation after 40—60 seconds.

In the choroidal vascular system and cilioretinal arteries, fluorescein shows up shortly before or simultaneously with the early retinal arterial phase. Normally, the dye has disappeared from the choroidal vascular system in the retinal venous phase, while some fluorescence usually persists from the choroidal tissue for about 10 minutes.

In pathological conditions, fluorescein angiography may reveal changes in the retinal blood circulation, demonstrate leakage of dye from the vessels or may show characteristic fluorescein patterns, some of which may be of value in the differential diagnosis of various fundus diseases.

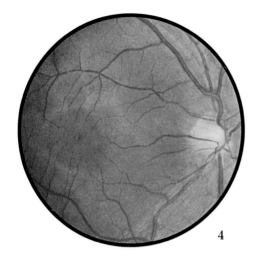

4

*Right eye. Normal fundus in a Negro.*

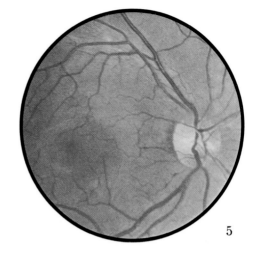

5

*Right eye. Normal fundus in an Indian.*

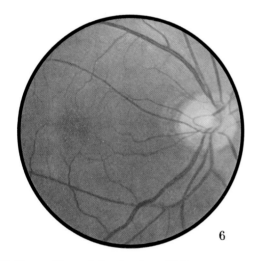

6

*Right eye. Normal fundus in a Chinese.*

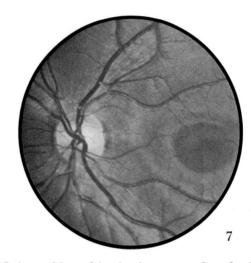

7

*Left eye. Normal fundus in a young Greenlander.*

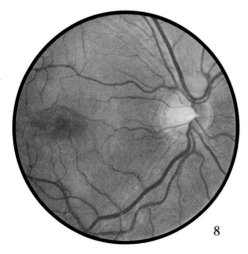

8

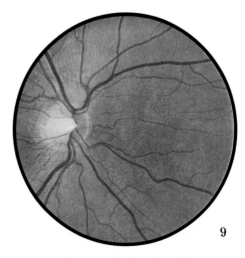

9

*Figures 8 and 9. Right eye. Temporal and nasal part of the same fundus. The fundus shows* *marked tessellation. The fundus color corresponds to a dark-haired person.*

# Albinism
## (Figures 12—13)

Albinism is a congenital and hereditary defect, due to an inhibition of pigment development. It may involve all pigmented structures including the hair, skin or eyes, but this is rare. More often the condition is incomplete, showing a deficiency of pigment in various structures or involving the eyes alone. In the last condition, called ocular albinism, the rest of the body is normally or lightly pigmented.

General albinism is inherited as an autosomal, recessive trait, while ocular albinism is usually sex-linked, affecting the males through female carriers.

Albinism is frequently accompanied by photophobia, nystagmus, amblyopia and considerable errors of refraction. The irides are pink-gray and translucent and the pupil is red.

OPHTHALMOSCOPICALLY, the fundus is orange-yellow (Fig. 13) and the macular area has a pink tint (Fig. 12). The foveal and macular reflexes are absent (Fig. 12). The choroidal vessels are seen plainly. The retinal vessels and the disc are normal (Fig. 13).

The condition is very characteristic and should not be confused with pseudoalbinism.

HISTOPATHOLOGICALLY, the retina and the choroid show no or only small amounts of pigment, and a real fovea is often lacking.

# Carriers of Albinism
## (Figures 14—15)

In ocular albinism, which is usually sex-linked, female carriers frequently show characteristic morphological fundus changes. However, visual disturbances are not present.

OPHTHALMOSCOPICALLY, the fundus periphery shows coarse pigmentation and depigmentation (Figs. 14—15), in some places assuming a salt-and-pepper appearance. The pigmentation diminishes in the macular direction. The disc and the retinal vessels are normal.

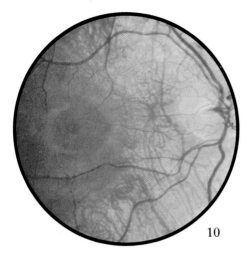

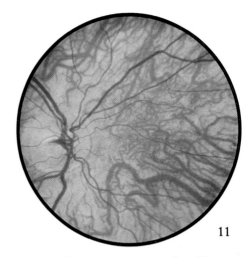

Figures 10 and 11. Right eye. Temporal and nasal part of the same pseudoalbinotic fundus.

The fundus has an orange-red color. The macular area has a normal appearance.

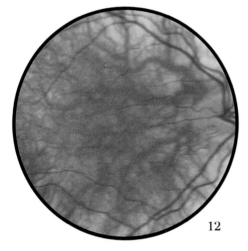

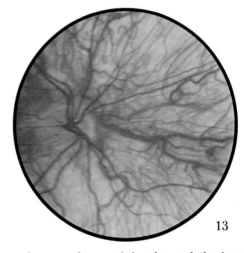

Figures 12 and 13. Right eye. Temporal and nasal part of the same albinotic fundus. The

macular area has a pink color and the fovea is absent.

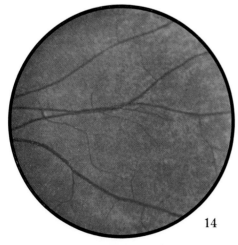

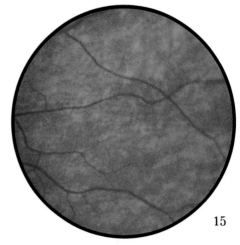

Right eye. Carrier of albinism. Coarse pigmentation in fundus periphery.

Right eye. Carrier of albinism. Depigmentation in fundus periphery.

# Medullated Nerve Fibers
### (Figures 16—21)

The normal centrifugal myelinization of the optic nerve fibers usually stops at the lamina cribrosa. Sometimes, however, myelinization continues into the retina for a variable distance. Medullated nerve fibers are never present at birth, but may develop during the first few months of postnatal life. Once developed, the medullated nerve fibers remain unchanged throughout life, except in cases where an atrophic process of the optic nerve supervenes, in which case they gradually disappear.

Vision is seldom affected in this condition unless the macula is involved. However, macular involvement is rare. There is usually a scotoma which is slightly smaller than the corresponding opaque area in the fundus.

The condition is rather common. It is usually unilateral, but may occur bilaterally.

OPHTHALMOSCOPICALLY, medullated nerve fibers are seen as whitish, brilliant-white or yellowish-white, opaque, silky patches with a finely striated surface and a feathered margin (Figs. 16—19). Most frequently, the patches are tongue-shaped or flame-shaped and situated at the upper or lower margin of the disc (Fig. 16), but size and shape vary widely (Figs. 16, 18—21). Occasionally, the medullated fibers surround the disc (Figs. 18 and 20) or the macular area (Fig. 19). Rarely, they involve the macular area (Fig. 21) or lie as isolated patches in the fundus periphery (Fig. 17). The retinal vessels are partly or completely obscured by the medullated fibers in the opaque area.

The ophthalmoscopic picture of medullated nerve fibers is very characteristic, and should not be confused with woolly exudates, acute juxtapapillary choroiditis, optic atrophy or retinal branch artery occlusion.

HISTOPATHOLOGICALLY, myelinated nerve fibers are found corresponding to the opaque patches.

# Pits in the Optic Disc
### (Figures 22—23 and 377)

Pits or holes in the optic disc are not uncommon. The condition is generally considered to be a minimal, atypical coloboma and the defect is usually unilateral.

Pits in the optic disc are frequently present in cases of central serous retinopathy (Fig. 377).

The anomaly usually causes no visual

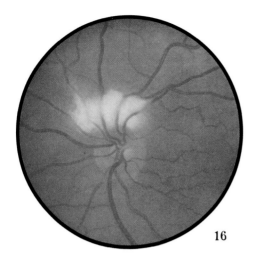

16

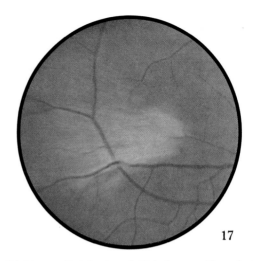

17

*Left eye. Medullated nerve fibers situated just above the optic disc.*

*Right eye. Patch of medullated nerve fibers in the fundus periphery.*

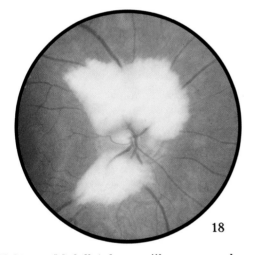

18

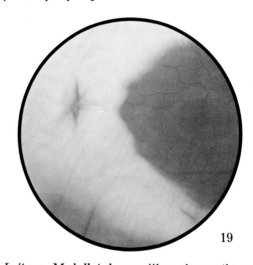

19

*Right eye. Medullated nerve fibers surround and partly obscure the optic disc.*

*Left eye. Medullated nerve fibers obscure the optic disc. Macular area free.*

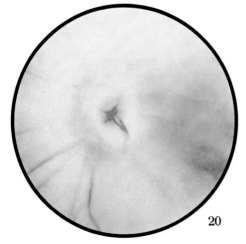

20

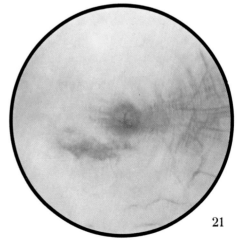

21

*Figures 20 and 21. Left eye. Disc and macular area of the same fundus. Extensive area of*

*medullated nerve fibers in the posterior pole.*

disturbances, but if the papillomacular bundle is involved, central vision may be gravely affected. The visual field usually shows enlargement of the blind spot or sector-shaped defects, sometimes producing a partial or complete paracentral or central scotoma.

OPHTHALMOSCOPICALLY, the pit is usually seen as a small vertically oval, sharply defined depression at the temporal side of the disc (Figs. 22—23). The base of the pit may be seen clearly or may be covered by grayish-white tissue. Some pigment accumulation may also be present.

HISTOPATHOLOGICALLY, the lamina cribrosa is defective, corresponding to the pit, and the defective area is partially filled with glial tissue.

# Colobomas of the Fundus
### (Figures 24—27)

Colobomas may involve the eyelid, iris, ciliary body, lens, choroid, retina, and the optic nerve head. Typical bulbar colobomas are the result of imperfect closure of the fetal ocular cleft. They may be complete, involving all the bulbar structures associated with the embryonic cleft, or partial, when the defect is less extensive. Typical colobomas are situated in the lower nasal region of the eye, atypical elsewhere. Typical colobomas are often bilateral, while atypical are usually unilateral.

Central vision is frequently reduced, although the macula may appear normal ophthalmoscopically. In the visual field there is a scotoma corresponding to the coloboma, although usually smaller than the defective area. Strabismus and nystagmus are common in this condition.

OPHTHALMOSCOPICALLY, a fundus coloboma is seen as a sharply defined, whitish or grayish-white area of variable extension, and usually situated below the disc (Figs. 26—27).

It is frequently bridged by a few retinal and some choroidal vessels (Fig. 26) and bordered by some pigment deposits (Figs. 25—27). In the colobomatous area the sclera may appear ectatic (Fig. 27). Colobomas are usually single, but several colobomas may be present in the same fundus. The defect may also involve the disc (Fig. 24). In these cases, the disc is seen as a shallow or deep grayish-white cavity, and the cavity is filled with varying amounts of whitish glial tissue.

Fundus colobomas, even the small ones, are very typical and should not be confused with chorioretinal scars, which sometimes may assume an appearance resembling small isolated colobomas.

HISTOPATHOLOGICALLY, typical fundal colobomas are characterized by localized defects in the retina and choroid. The defective retina may be represented by a thin membrane containing scattered retinal elements and the choroid by some mesodermal remnants, while Bruch's membrane is absent. The sclera is often abnormally thin and somewhat ectatic. If the optic disc is involved, the coloboma may be represented by a mass of poorly developed glial and neural tissue at the disc.

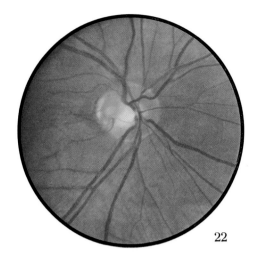

22

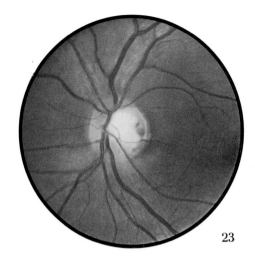

23

*Right eye. Small crater-like hole in the temporal part of the optic disc.*

*Left eye. Small pigmented crater-like hole in the temporal part of the optic disc.*

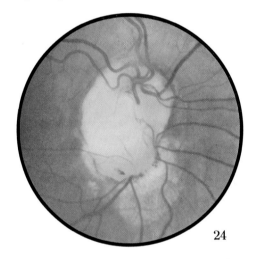

24

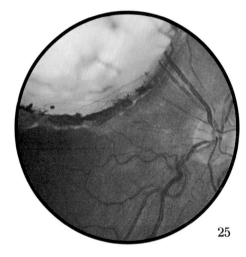

25

*Right eye. Incomplete coloboma of the optic disc and the choroid.*

*Right eye. Choroidal and retinal coloboma in the upper temporal quadrant.*

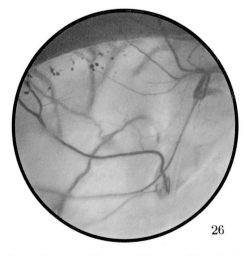

26

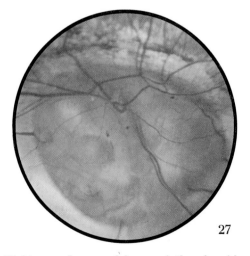

27

*Left eye. Large coloboma of the choroid and retina in the lower half of the fundus.*

*Right eye. Large coloboma of the choroid and retina in the lower half of the fundus.*

# Congenital Macular Cyst
(Figures 28—29)

A congenital macular cyst is a rare condition, but constitutes a well-defined clinical entity. It may occur sporadically, affecting one or both eyes, or be transmitted hereditarily. In the latter case, the condition is possibly identical with the infantile type of heredomacular degeneration (Best's type).

In early stages vision is only slightly affected, and much less than should be expected from the fundal lesion. During middle age, however, visual disturbances usually develop and eventually central vision is lost.

OPHTHALMOSCOPICALLY, the congenital macular cyst, also named vitelliform macular cyst, is seen as a pale, rounded, slightly elevated patch in the macular area (Figs. 28 and 29). The evolution of the lesion is exceedingly slow. Finally, however, the lesion is converted into an atrophic scar with or without pigmentation.

# Epipapillary Membrane and Bergmeister's Papilla
(Figures 30—31)

Throughout the greater part of embryonic life the hyaloid artery and some of the major retinal vessels are sheathed by cells originating from the primitive epithelial papilla of Bergmeister. Shortly before birth, the hyaloid artery and its sheaths atrophy.

Sometimes, however, remnants of the sheath may remain on the disc, either sheathing the retinal vessels for a short distance (Fig. 30) or persisting as a well-defined membrane or web of opaque tissue, the epipapillary membrane, stretching over the optic disc (Fig. 30) or even presenting a more solid, prominent mass of tissue in front of the disc (Fig. 31), known as Bergmeister's papilla. This mass, which may be very prominent at birth and during infancy, often projects several diopters into the vitreous, and frequently has a tendency to reduce in size while the child is growing up.

In the differential diagnosis persistent primary vitreous, retinoblastoma and angiomatosis of the retina have to be considered.

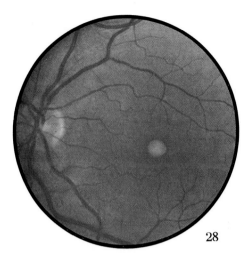

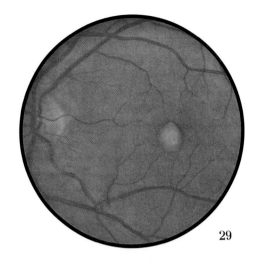

28

29

*Left eye. Small, round, yellowish vitelliform cyst in the macular area.*

*Left eye. Small, oval, yellowish vitelliform cyst in the macular area.*

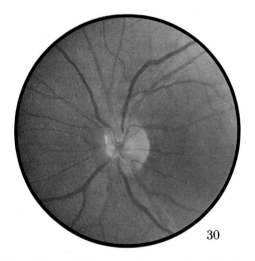

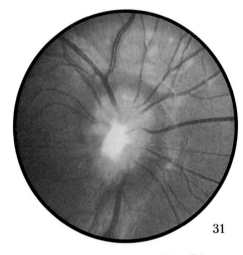

30

31

*Left eye. Epipapillary membrane on the optic disc.*

*Right eye. Bergmeister's papilla. Disc covered with a web of opaque tissue.*

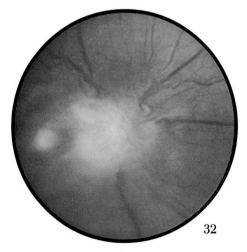

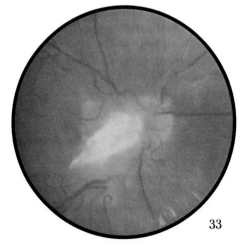

32

33

*Right eye. Persistent hyperplastic primary vitreous.*

*Same eye as figure 32, two years later. The whitish tissue has diminished in size.*

# Persistent Hyperplastic Primary Vitreous
### (Figures 32—36)

Persistent hyperplastic primary vitreous is rare. It is usually characterized by a hyperplastic membrane covering a smaller or larger part of the posterior surface of the lens, but at times the preretinal changes may be more obvious than those behind the lens. In these cases, prepapillary (Figs. 32—33) or preretinal veils or masses of whitish tissue (Figs. 34—35) are present together with remnants of the hyaloid artery (Fig. 36).

The condition may also be related to congenital retinal detachment with falciform retinal folds.

# Retrolental Fibroplasia
### (Figures 37—39)

Retrolental fibroplasia is a condition occurring especially in premature infants, but it may also occur, although rarely, in full-term children.

The condition is usually seen in premature infants who have been placed in a highly oxygenated incubator or who have received oxygen in high concentration by other methods.

The condition becomes evident ophthalmoscopically usually five to ten weeks after removal from the high oxygen level, and is nearly always bilateral.

In cases of retrolental fibroplasia, vision is almost invariably decreased and blindness often occurs in the cicatricial phase. In addition to the ocular symptoms, neurological symptoms and mental retardation occur in a high percentage of cases.

OPHTHALMOSCOPIC APPEARANCE: When the premature infant with his immature retinal vascular system is exposed to a high oxygen level, the retinal vessels and especially the arteries become narrowed or even obliterated. When the infant is later exposed to a normal oxygen level which means that the retina is now suffering from relative anoxia, the retinal vessels may react with venous fullness (Fig. 39) and later with a disorganized new vessel formation, especially in the fundus periphery. Together with this new vessel formation, a certain amount of fibrous tissue is developed. If not too extensive, these fibrous formations may remain as isolated patches, but the fibrous tissue formation usually continues, leading to traction in the retina within the first year of life. This causes retinal de-

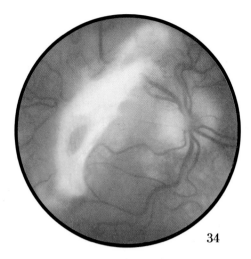

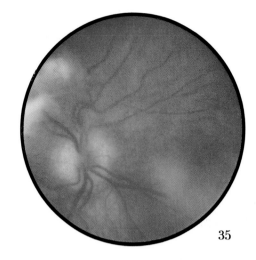

*Figures 34 and 35. Right eye. Temporal and nasal part of the same fundus. Persistent* *hyperplastic primary vitreous. Whitish fibrous tissue projects far into the vitreous.*

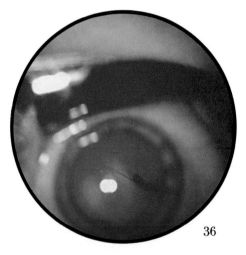

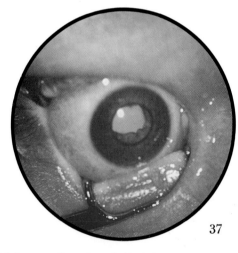

*Right eye. Persistent hyaloid artery attached to the lens by a foot-plate.*

*Right eye. Retrolental fibroplasia with annular retrolental fibrous mass.*

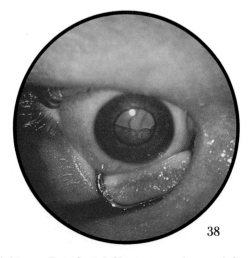

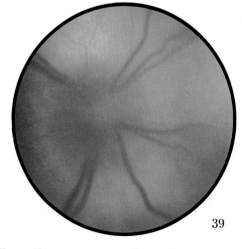

*Right eye. Retrolental fibrous mass is seen below, detached retina above.*

*From the same eye as figure 38. Flat retinal detachment.*

tachment (Figs. 37—39) and eventually the formation of a retrolental fibrous membrane, resulting in microphthalmos or phthisis of the globe.

In the differential diagnosis, retinoblastoma and congenital malformations of the eye have to be considered. At a late stage congenital falciform detachment is often impossible to distinguish from a not fully developed retrolental fibroplasia.

HISTOPATHOLOGICALLY, the condition is characterized by the formation of new-formed vessels, which at the early stage are limited to the retinal surface, but later are present together with fibrous tissue formation in the vitreous. Later still, the condition shows detachment of the retina due to traction and eventually the formation of a dense sheath of retrolental fibrous tissue, producing a retrolental membrane.

# Falciform Retinal Detachment
## (Figures 40—41)

Falciform retinal detachment is frequently bilateral, and is typically associated with the persistance of remnants of the hyaloid artery. In most cases the condition is due to developmental arrest, but in some cases it must be regarded as an abortive form of retrolental fibroplasia.

Visual acuity may be reduced or even damaged severely as the process usually occurs in the lower temporal quadrant and may show some extension into the macular area.

OPHTHALMOSCOPICALLY, the falciform detachment is usually seen as a broad retinal fold extending from the disc into the far fundus periphery (Figs. 40—41), but folds may also commence elsewhere in the fundus. In most cases the fundus appears quite normal apart from the retinal fold (Fig. 41), but sometimes the retina appears very thin or absent, giving the impression of looking straight into the choroid (Fig. 40). In these cases, only few retinal vessels may be encountered. Remnants of the hyaloid artery are usually present, and the condition is usually stationary.

HISTOPATHOLOGICALLY, the retina is pulled inwards and the whole retina may show some dysplasia, suggesting a disturbance of growth of the inner layer of the optic cup. Retinal rosettes may be present, but the retinal pigment epithelium is unaffected.

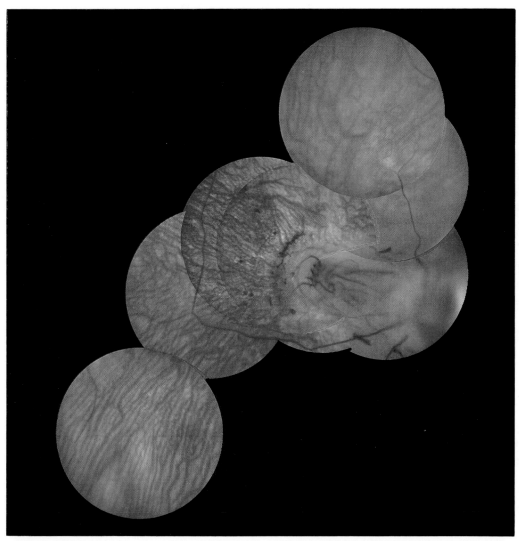

*Figure 40. Composite picture. Left eye. Falciform retinal detachment. An elevated fold of retinal* tissue extends from the optic disc to the lower temporal fundus periphery.

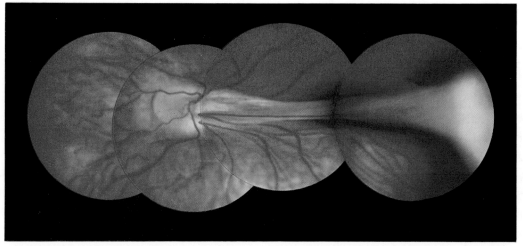

*Figure 41. Composite picture. Left eye. Falciform retinal fold emerging from the optic disc to the* periphery of the lower temporal quadrant where it is attached to the ciliary body.

# Fundus Changes in Myopia
### (Figures 42—53)

Clinically, cases of myopia may be divided into two groups, simple myopia and excessive or malignant myopia.

Simple myopia is a physiological variation in refraction, usually appearing in children of school-age. When demonstrated it seldom exceeds a few diopters. Although the myopia may increase half a diopter or more annually over a period of years, progression always stops at adolescence, and good vision is maintained with suitable correction throughout life.

The fundus may be normal, tessellated or show a myopic crescent at the temporal side of the disc, or it may be lightly pigmented, or even pseudoalbinotic.

OPHTHALMOSCOPICALLY, early cases of simple myopia may show no fundus changes, but later myopic crescent or conus formation usually becomes apparent as a whitish crescent outside the scleral ring at the temporal side of the disc (Figs. 43—45). The crescent is frequently bordered temporally by some pigment. The fundus color is frequently uniform, but tessellation or lightly pigmented areas may occur (Fig. 42), except in the macular area, and the retinal vessels appear normal.

Excessive or malignant myopia occurs at all ages and may be present even at birth. In this condition there is usually progressive elongation of the posterior segment of the eye, excessive increase in the myopia and a development of degenerative changes in the fundus. Visual acuity is reduced in spite of correction of the error of refraction.

The fundus changes include myopic crescent, disseminated choroidal atrophies, macular degeneration and cystoid degeneration in the fundus periphery, and the changes may occur singly or together.

OPHTHALMOSCOPICALLY, excessive or malignant myopia almost always shows a myopic crescent of varying size (Fig. 45)

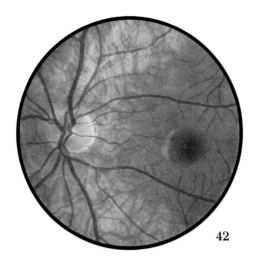

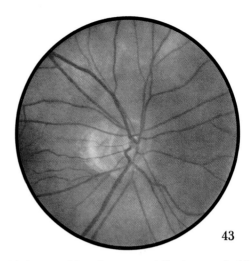

*Left eye. Fundus in simple myopia, from a blond person.*

*Right eye. Myopic conus at the temporal side of the disc.*

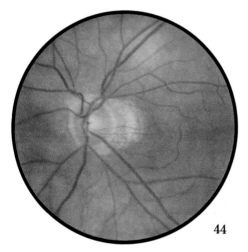

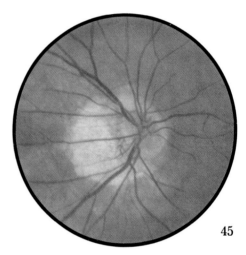

*Left eye. Myopic conus at the temporal side of the disc.*

*Right eye. Large myopic conus at the temporal side of the disc.*

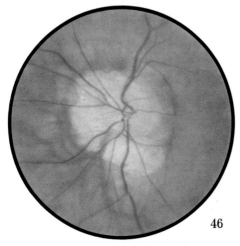

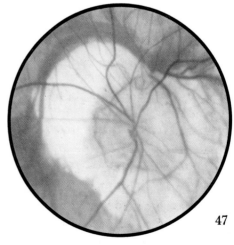

*Left eye. Peripapillary atrophy in excessive myopia.*

*Right eye. Large peripapillary atrophy in excessive myopia.*

or more extensive peripapillary atrophy (Figs. 46—47). The fundus color may vary widely, ranging from the normal red color (Figs. 48—50) to an orange color (Fig. 53). The latter is seen in quasi-albinotic cases where the choroidal vessels are seen plainly and the choroidal intervascular spaces appear enlarged. The retinal vessels appear slightly narrower than in the normal fundus.

In the course of time, disseminated choroidal atrophies may occur (Figs. 51—52). They are seen as sharply defined, more or less confluent white or yellowish-white patches of variable size and shape, often accompanied by some irregular, patchy pigmentation.

At times, macular changes develop. They often start quite suddenly with subretinal or deep retinal hemorrhages (Figs. 48—50) accompanied by some macular edema. The hemorrhages and the edema are absorbed slowly and may ultimately be replaced by organized exudate, an atrophic chorioretinal scar (Fig. 52) or a mass of nearly black pigment (Fig. 51). The latter is known as Fuchs' spot.

In the fundus periphery, besides small pigmented spots and depigmented patches, cystoid degeneration often appears in girdles which run concentrically or lie in irregular nests. The cystoid degeneration gives the fundus periphery a fine, honeycombed appearance. In time, the cystic spaces enlarge. Vitreous adhesions, together with increased mobility of the vitreous due to liquefaction and perhaps trauma, may convert the cystic spaces into holes; in some cases this may be a factor in the development of retinal detachment.

HISTOPATHOLOGICALLY, a myopic crescent is formed at the temporal side of the disc by the lack of retinal pigment epithelium, Bruch's membrane and choroid, the latter defect being usually the smallest. The myopic atrophy in the fundus is characterized by changes in the choroid and the retina. The choroid is thinned, stroma pigment is reduced and the choroidal vessels diminished in number, especially in the choriocapillaris, which is atrophic. The elastic part of Bruch's membrane is thinned and holes develop. The retina shows varying degrees of atrophy and cystoid degeneration.

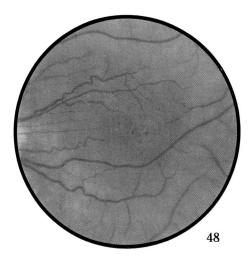

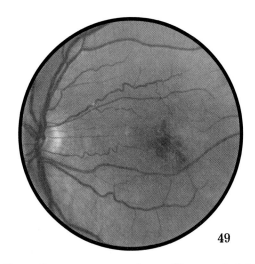

48

49

*Left eye. Incipient development of Fuchs' spot in excessive myopia.*

*From the same eye as figure 48, a week later. Macular hemorrhage increased.*

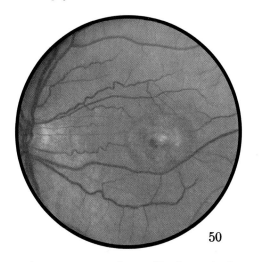

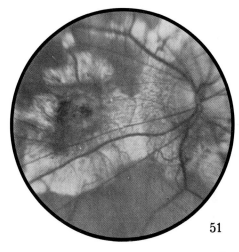

50

51

*From the same eye as figure 49, six weeks later. Pigmented scar is developing.*

*Right eye. Disseminated myopic atrophy. A Fuchs' spot seen in the macula.*

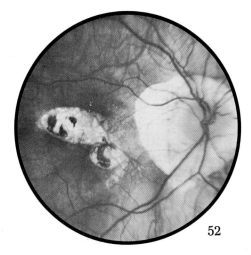

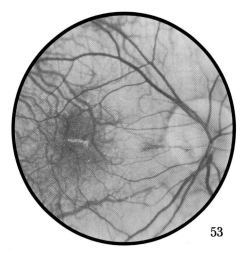

52

53

*Right eye. Excessive myopia with atrophies and scattered pigmentation.*

*Right eye. Excessive myopic, quasi-albinotic fundus with temporal conus.*

# The Optic Disc

## Physiological Variations and Congenital Abnormalities.
### (Figures 54—78)

The optic disc is the most obvious feature in the ophthalmoscopic view of the fundus. It measures about 1.5 mm in diameter and corresponds in position with the entrance of the optic nerve into the bulb.

OPHTHALMOSCOPICALLY, the optic disc is seen as a pale, well-defined, round (Fig. 54) or vertically slightly oval disc (Figs. 55—59) with a pink or yellowish-red tint which contrasts notably with the color of the fundus. The nasal part of the disc is often slightly redder than the temporal part (Fig. 54). The retinal vessels usually make their appearance at the nasal side of the center of the optic disc. At the temporal side of the entering vessels, the disc usually shows a central depression. This physiological excavation may be shallow (Fig. 58) or deep (Fig. 59), small (Figs. 54—55) or large (Fig. 60), but it never occupies the full extent of the optic disc.

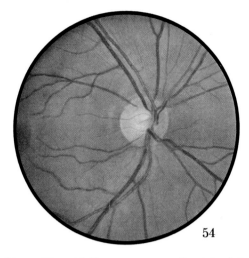

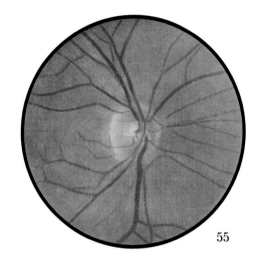

*Right eye. Normal disc, seen as a yellowish-pink, well-defined round area.*

*Right eye. Normal disc. The disc is slightly more red nasally than temporally.*

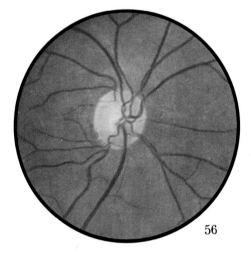

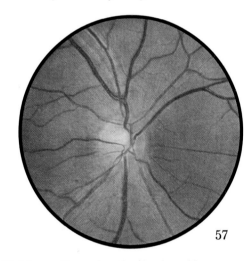

*Right eye. Normal optic disc and tessellated fundus.*

*Right eye. Normal optic disc in a Negro.*

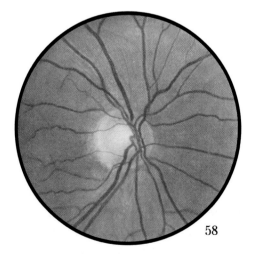

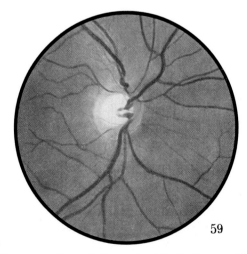

*Right eye. Normal optic disc with temporal physiological excavation.*

*Right eye. Central, deep physiological excavation of the optic disc.*

The central excavation is lighter than the surrounding part of the disc, and when deep, the lamina cribrosa may be visible in its base. Although the optic disc usually measures about 1.5 mm in diameter, it may show wide variations from very small (Figs. 61—62) to very large (Figs. 63—64). In old people, a large disc may be simulated by the occurrence of massive peripapillary atrophy (senile peripapillary atrophy) (Fig. 65).

The optic disc is frequently bordered by two more or less complete rings. The outer, the choroidal ring, is pigmented (Figs. 67—69) and the inner, the scleral ring, is whitish (Figs. 60, 70—71).

In rare instances, the disc may assume a grayish-red color due to pigment accumulation on the disc (Fig. 66), or it may even appear slate-gray or nearly black (papilla grisea).

Conus formation is a rather common

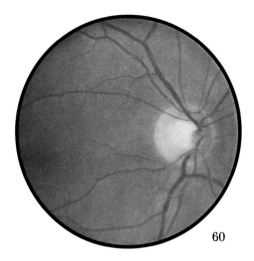

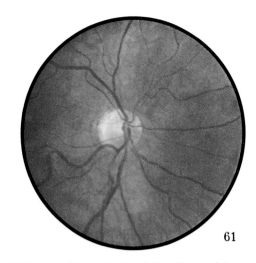

*Right eye. Normal disc with large temporal physiological excavation.*

*Right eye. Hypoplasia of the disc and temporal conus.*

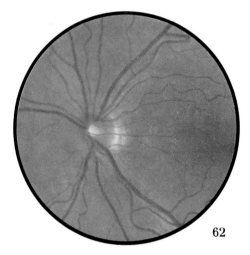

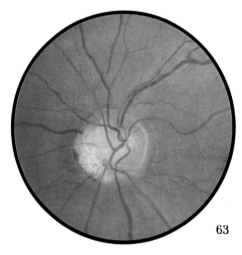

*Left eye. Small, pink optic disc. Normal physiological variation.*

*Left eye. Large optic disc with conus formation nasally.*

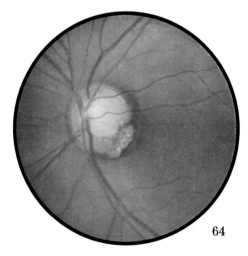

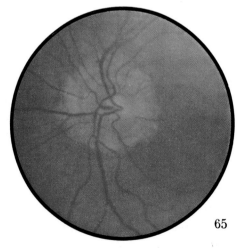

*Left eye. Large optic disc with conus formation and some pigmentation.*

*Left eye. Senile peripapillary atrophy.*

occurrence, especially in myopic eyes. The condition may be divided into temporal conus, which is the most frequent, nasal conus and inferior conus.

Temporal conus or crescent is seen as a whitish crescent outside the scleral ring at the temporal side of the disc, and is most often found in association with myopia (Figs. 43—45).

Nasal conus or crescent is seen as a whitish crescent at the nasal side of the disc (Figs. 72—74) and the condition is often accompanied by some deformity of the disc. The disc is often slightly elevated temporally and shallowed nasally. The retinal vessels emerge from the temporal side of the disc, at first running nasally and then bending sharply when passing into the retina. This condition is often associated with myopia and a notable degree of astigmatism.

Inferior conus or crescent is a whitish

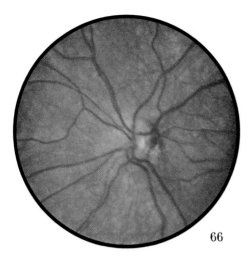

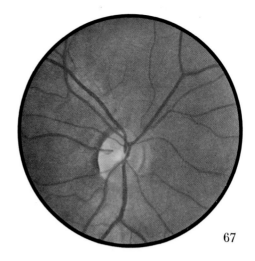

66

67

*Left eye. The optic disc is grayish and shows heavy pigment accumulation temporally.*

*Right eye. Normal optic disc with accumulation of choroidal pigment temporally.*

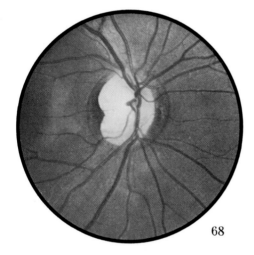

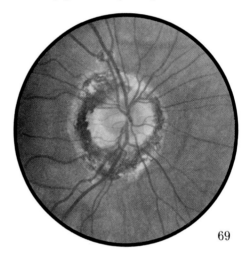

68

69

*Right eye. Large optic disc surrounded by a broad choroidal ring.*

*Right eye. The normal optic disc is surrounded by a broad choroidal ring.*

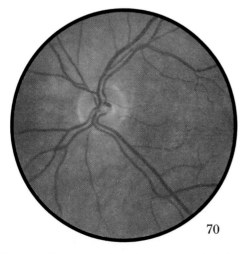

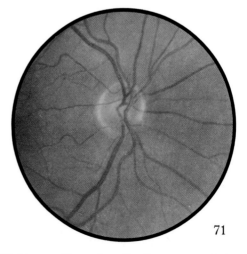

70

71

*Left eye. Normal optic disc surrounded by a yellowish-white scleral ring.*

*Right eye. Normal optic disc surrounded by a yellowish-white scleral ring.*

crescent situated just below the disc (Figs. 75—77) and often accompanied by some deformity of the disc. It is most often seen in myopic eyes and especially in those exhibiting a notable degree of astigmatism. Inferior conus is considered to be a developmental defect, a kind of incomplete coloboma.

In rare instances, the physiological optic cup and the whole surface of the disc may be covered by a delicate web of glial tissue (Fig. 78), which may give the disc an appearance of swelling, but just as in pseudopapilledema, venous engorgement, hemorrhages and exudates are never present.

The condition Membrana epipapillaris and Bergmeister's papilla are discussed elsewhere.

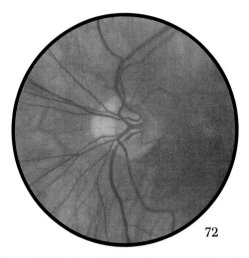

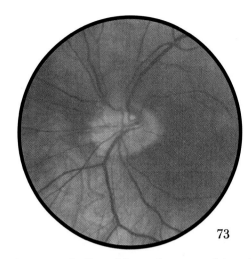

*Left eye. Optic disc with nasal conus and inverted vascular trunk.*

*Left eye. Optic disc with nasal conus and inverted vascular trunk.*

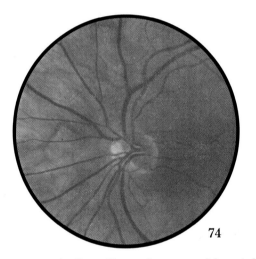

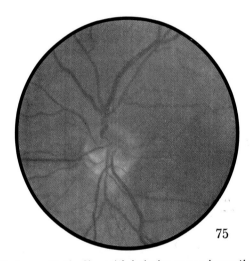

*Left eye. Optic disc with nasal conus and inverted vascular trunk.*

*Left eye. Optic disc with inferior conus formation.*

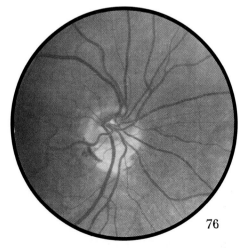

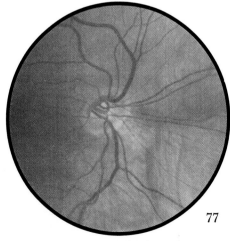

*Right eye. Optic disc with inferior conus formation.*

*Right eye. Optic disc with inferior conus formation.*

# Pseudopapilledema
(Figures 79—83)

Pseudopapilledema or pseudoneuritis is a rare congenital variation most often observed in small, hypermetropic eyes or in eyes with hypermetropic astigmatism.

The condition is stationary and visual disturbances are seldom present.

OPHTHALMOSCOPICALLY, it is characterized by swelling of the disc, which is slightly reddened, the margin having a blurred appearance and the disc projecting forward, but seldom more than a few diopters (Fig. 79). The retinal vessels are of normal caliber. Venous engorgement, hemorrhages and exudates are never present. The condition is sometimes associated with drusen of the optic disc, which will be discussed separately (Figs. 80—83).

The condition is of importance as it may be confused with papilledema. In the differential diagnosis, fluorescein angiography may be of value. In papilledema, there is usually a leakage of dye from the disc. In pseudopapilledema the angiogram is always normal. In the earliest stages of papilledema, however, the angiogram may also be normal. Normal fluorescein angiography therefore does not exclude papilledema, and repeated angiography may be necessary to exclude papilledema. The conditions can also be differentiated by observation over a period of the non-progressive nature and absence of vascular changes in pseudopapilledema.

# Drusen of the Optic Disc
(Figures 80—83)

Drusen of the optic disc is a rare hereditary condition inherited as an irregular dominant trait and unrelated to colloid bodies in Bruch's membrane. Drusen of the optic disc may be observed at any age and the condition is frequently bilateral.

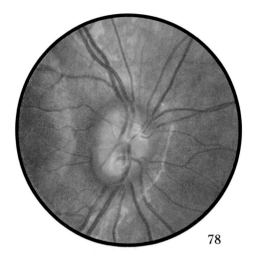

78

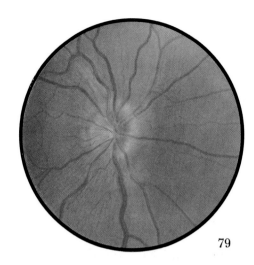

79

*Right eye. Congenital anomaly. Disc covered by a delicate web of glial tissue.*

*Right eye. Pseudopapilledema. The disc margin is blurred nasally.*

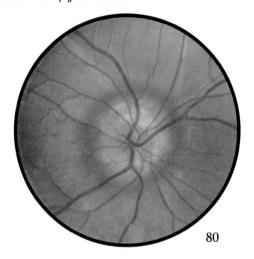

80

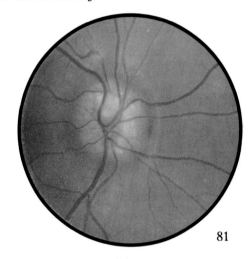

81

*Right eye. Pseudopapilledema and drusen of the disc.*

*Right eye. Pseudopapilledema and drusen of the disc.*

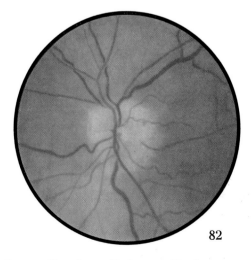

82

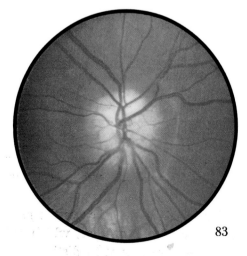

83

*Left eye. Pseudopapilledema with drusen embedded in the optic nerve tissue.*

*Right eye. Pseudopapilledema with drusen embedded in the optic nerve tissue.*

There are usually no or only slight visual disturbances, but the blind spot may be enlarged, and sectorial or irregular scotomas may result from nerve fiber degeneration. In rare instances, the visual field shows a concentric constriction.

OPHTHALMOSCOPICALLY, drusen of the optic disc are seen as small white or yellowish-white, glistening, spherical or grain-like depositis, situated superficially (Figs. 80—81) or deeply (Figs. 82—83) in the optic disc tissue. They often lie in groups either at the periphery of the disc or centrally. The disc margin is more or less blurred and the disc often shows an apparent increase in size, especially if the drusen are situated deep in the optic nerve head. They may also cause prominence of the optic disc and mimic papilledema.

In cases with blurred margins and elevation of the optic disc, the condition has to be distinguished from papilledema and papillitis. Occasionally, the condition may mimic an optic atrophy.

In the differential diagnosis, fluorescein angiography is valuable because drusen of the optic disc often show a characteristic fluorescein pattern.

HISTOPATHOLOGICALLY, drusen of the optic disc are seen as laminated, homogeneous, acellular masses, usually containing calcareous concretions and situated within the substance of the optic disc.

# Papilledema
(Figures 84—102, 136, 185—188, 192 and 222—225)

Papilledema is a non-inflammatory swelling of the optic nerve head or disc. It is an important ophthalmoscopic sign in different intracranial, ocular, neural and orbital conditions, as well as in some systemic diseases.

In the vast majority of cases the papilledema named choked disc, which ophthalmoscopically cannot be distinguished from papilledema of other origin, is due to brain tumors. This papilledema is more frequently present in subtentorial than supratentorial conditions. Tumors localized to the region of the corpora quadrigemina, pineal body, fourth ventricle and cerebellum often produce papilledema. Pituitary tumors, however, rarely produce papilledema. Occasionally, tumors of the olfactory or frontal lobe, or the sphenoidal ridge may cause optic atrophy on the same side and papilledema on the opposite side (Foster-Kennedy syndrome).

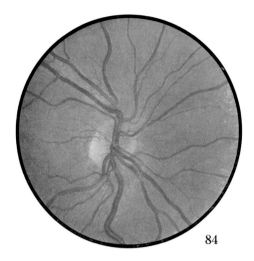

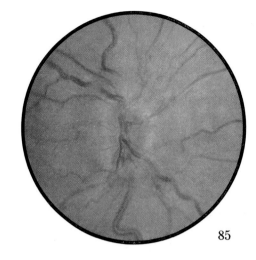

84

85

*Right eye. Normal optic disc.*

*The same eye as figure 84, four years later. Papilledema in cerebellar tumor, early stage.*

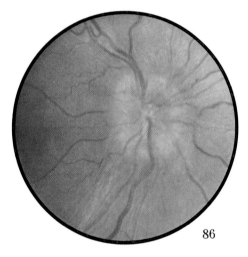

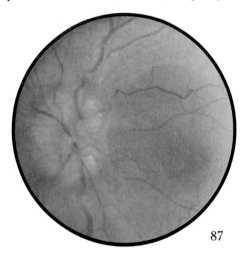

86

87

*Figures 86 and 87. Right and left eyes. Papilledema due to an ethmoidal meningeoma, early*

*stage. The discs project about one to two diopters.*

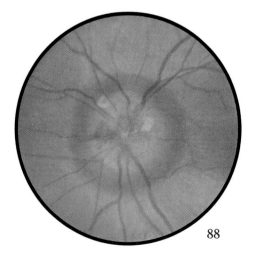

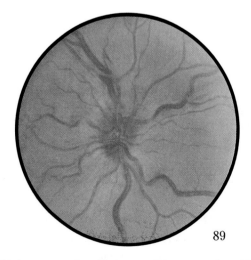

88

89

*Left eye. Slight papilledema in a pseudopapilledema disc with drusen.*

*Right eye. Papilledema due to sphenoidal meningeoma. Disc projects one diopter.*

Chiasma arachnoiditis may sometimes give rise to a similar ophthalmoscopic picture (Pseudo Foster-Kennedy syndrome—Figs. 102—103).

Papilledema may also be observed in such conditions as brain abcesses, cerebral metastases (Figs. 90—91), meningitis, sinus thrombosis (Fig. 93), intracranial hemorrhage (Fig. 92), hydrocephalus, premature cranial synostosis, cerebral syphilis (Fig. 100) and tuberculosis; in tumors of the optic nerve, in orbital tumors (Fig. 101), cysts and vascular abnormalities; in central retinal venous thrombosis (Figs. 222—225); in congenital heart disease (Fig. 136); in leukemia (Fig. 97), severe anemia, polycythemia, dysproteinemia (Figs. 98—99), and malignant hypertension (Figs. 96, 185—188, 192).

The papilledema named choked disc and papilledema in systemic diseases are usually bilateral, although the degree of swelling may differ on the two sides. Papilledema in ocular, orbital and neural conditions, however, is usually unilateral.

Papilledema usually develops slowly in the course of weeks or months. Occasionally, for example in traumatic intracranial hemorrhage, it may develop in the course of a few hours.

For a long period there may be no symptoms at all or only short attacks of hazy vision or even momentary blindness (obscurations) lasting from to 10 to 30 seconds. At this stage, the blind spot is enlarged, but the vision and the peripheral visual field are intact unless the basic disorder causes field defects.

Long-standing papilledema sooner or later leads to optic atrophy. When atrophy develops, there is progressive contraction of the visual field and reduction of vision even to blindness.

OPHTHALMOSCOPICALLY, the disc in the early stages of papilledema is slightly redder than normal (compare Figs. 84 and 85) owing to a dilatation of the capil-

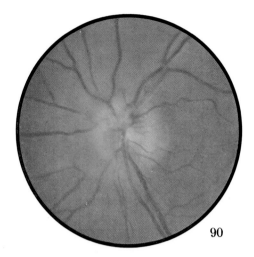

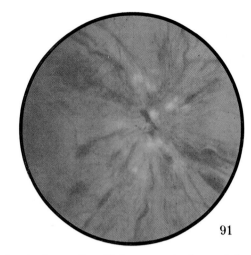

90

91

*Figures 90 and 91. Left and right eyes. Papill-edema due to hypernephroma metastases in both*

*hemispheres. Papilledema most advanced in the right eye.*

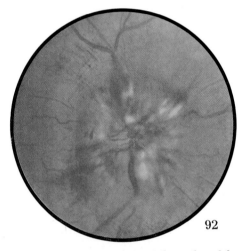

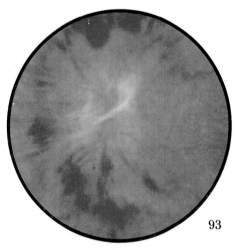

92

93

*Right eye. Papilledema in bilateral subdural hematoma, advanced stage.*

*Left eye. Chronic papilledema in sinus cavernosus thrombosis.*

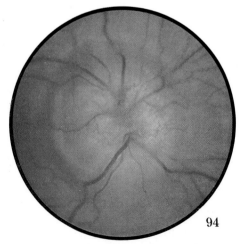

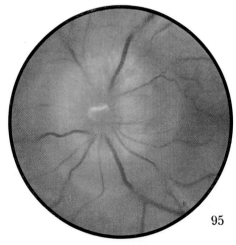

94

95

*Figures 94 and 95. Right and left eyes. Chronic papilledema in glioma of the frontal lobe. Both*

*discs enlarged and pale due to edema and gliosis, and project about four diopters.*

laries within the substance of the optic disc. The disc margin is slightly blurred, at first above and below, then nasally and finally temporally. The veins become congested (Fig. 89) and venous pulsation is almost always absent. The small vessels at the disc are dilated and seen more plainly than in the normal disc, and slight edema may fill the normal disc cup (Figs. 86—87).

When papilledema progresses into the fully developed stage, the increasing edema causes swelling and some pallor of the disc (Figs. 88, 90). The disc gradually projects forward from one (Figs. 86—89) to several diopters (Figs. 92, 98, 100), and may sometimes resemble a mushroom. The veins become engorged (Fig. 89), small splinter or flame-shaped hemorrhages and cotton-wool exudates appear at and around the disc (Figs. 91—93, 96, 97), fine light streaks indicating retinal edema radiate from the disc into the surrounding retina (Figs. 86—87),

and sometimes a macular star may develop. If the papilledema persists for some months glial proliferation may occur at the disc (Figs. 93—95).

If the basic disorder is removed or disappears, papilledema subsides, leaving no or only slight ophthalmoscopic traces.

In long-standing papilledema and in cases with persistent papilledema, chronic atrophic papilledema with optic atrophy develops. The edema gradually decreases and the disc becomes paler as a result of glial proliferation (Figs. 94—95). Finally, the disc appears grayish-white or white, flat or slightly cupped, the lamina cribrosa obscured by glial tissue, and the disc margin slightly ill-defined (Figs. 106—107, 111). Venous fullness disappears and the arteries become narrow.

The degree of pallor of the disc, however, often does not correspond with the degree of the functional loss.

It is not possible ophthalmoscopically to differentiate papilledema from acute

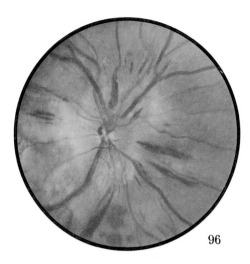

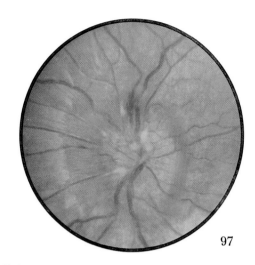

96

97

*Right eye. Papilledema in hypertensive neurore-tinopathy.*

*Left eye. Papilledema in leukemia. The disc projects about two diopters.*

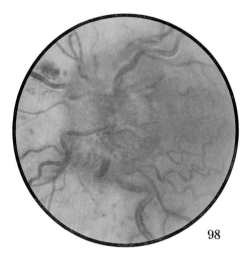

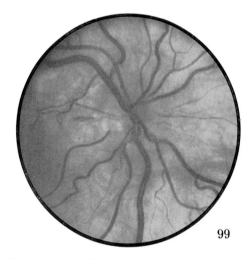

98

99

*Left eye. Chronic papilledema in macroglobuli-nemia.*

*Right eye. Papilledema in myelomatosis.*

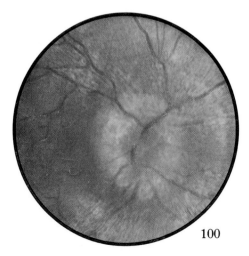

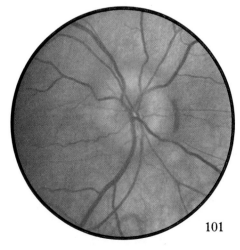

100

101

*Right eye. Chronic papilledema in neuroluetic infection.*

*Right eye. Slight papilledema due to a retrobulbar tumor.*

optic neuritis (papillitis). Clinically, the two conditions are distinguished by early loss of vision and presence of a central scotoma in optic neuritis.

Early stages of papilledema have to be distinguished from pseudopapilledema or pseudoneuritis. The distinction is almost impossible in a single ophthalmoscopy so that the patient has to be followed at short intervals. At times, fluorescein angiography may be of value in the differential diagnosis. A normal angiogram, however, does not exclude papilledema, while leakage of dye from the disc is characteristic of papilledema. Ophthalmoscopically, the conditions are differentiated by the continuous lack of venous engorgement, hemorrhages and exudates in pseudopapilledema. In the differential diagnosis, drusen of the optic disc has also to be considered. Papilledema should never be confused with occlusion of the central retinal vein or hypertensive neuroretinopathy.

HISTOPATHOLOGICALLY, papilledema is characterized by edema of the disc and the adjacent retina, swelling of the nerve fibers, engorgement of the veins, and frequently by hemorrhages and exudates.

# Atrophy of the Optic Nerve
### (Figures 103—113, 115—125, 301 and 435)

Optic atrophy is an irreversible degeneration of the optic nerve, and can be divided into the following three types: descending, ascending and post-inflammatory atrophy.

Descending optic atrophy is usually referred to as simple or "primary" atrophy, as there is no evidence of fundal disease, preceding papilledema or papillitis, but it also includes conditions such as tabetic (Fig. 435) and hereditary optic atrophy (Figs. 112—113), where the pathogenesis of the atrophy is not entirely clear. Descending or simple atrophy may follow retrobulbar neuritis in multiple sclerosis (Fig. 119), other demyelinating diseases (Fig. 110), intoxications, severe anemia, vascular disease (Figs. 108—109) including giant-cell arteritis, tumors in the optic nerve, tumors or hemorrhages compressing the optic nerve, traumatic lesions of the optic nerve, chiasma arachnoiditis (Fig. 103), and pituitary tumors (Fig. 107) or craniopharyngiomas (Figs. 104—105).

Ascending optic atrophy is secondary to retinal degeneration and inflammation. It occurs in conditions such as retinitis pigmentosa (Fig. 301) and glaucoma (Figs. 120—125, 161).

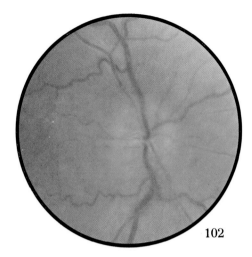

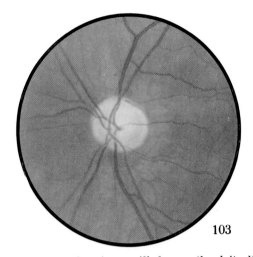

*Figures 102 and 103. Right and left eyes. Pseudo Foster-Kennedy syndrome. The right*   *disc shows chronic papilledema; the left disc is atrophic and slightly cupped.*

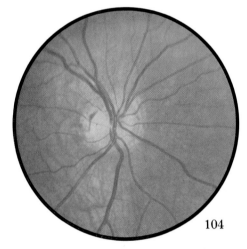

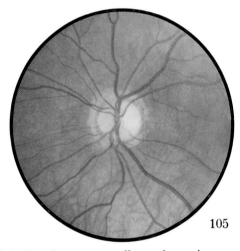

*Figures 104 and 105. Right and left eyes in craniopharyngeoma. The right disc is normal. The*   *left disc shows some pallor and cupping.*

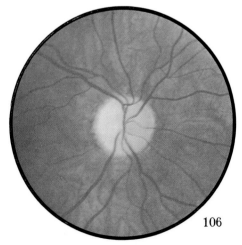

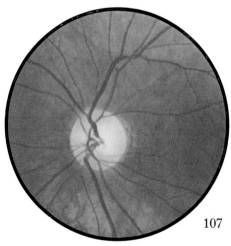

*Right eye. Optic nerve atrophy following chronic papilledema in cerebellar tumor.*   *Left eye. Optic nerve atrophy due to a pituitary tumor. Disc pale and slightly cupped.*

Post-inflammatory optic atrophy, usually referred to as "secondary" atrophy, may follow papilledema (Figs. 106, 111) or papillitis (Figs. 115—118).

In optic atrophy, vision is diminished and the visual field contracted to a varying degree. The diagnosis of optic atrophy, however, is more dependent on the loss of function than on the color of the disc, as we encounter cases with pallor of the disc in which no functional defect is present, and cases with functional defect but only slight pallor.

OPHTHALMOSCOPICALLY, the disc in descending or simple optic atrophy (Figs. 103, 105, 107—110, 112—113, 435) is sharply defined, pale, whitish or yellowish-white and shows a shallow saucer-shaped cupping. The lamina cribrosa is often seen plainly and without retraction of the base of the disc cup. The retinal vessels are narrow.

Following retrobulbar neuritis, there is usually only temporal sector-formed pallor of the disc (Fig. 119), with or without functional loss.

In ascending optic atrophy (Figs. 120—125, 161, 301), the disc is usually well-defined, pale, waxy-yellow or dirty-pink and slightly cupped, and the retinal vessels are narrow.

In post-inflammatory optic atrophy (Figs. 106, 111, 115—118), the disc is also pale, whitish or yellowish-white, but the margin is slightly irregular and there is no or only slight cupping of the disc, as glial tissue may fill the cup and sometimes continue along the retinal vessels for a short distance. The retinal vessels are narrow and peripapillary atrophy is usually present together with some pigmentation.

However, the ophthalmoscopic appearance of descending, ascending and post-inflammatory optic atrophy is often very similar, and it may be difficult or impossible to distinguish these conditions ophthalmoscopically.

It is, however, of importance to distinguish glaucomatous optic atrophy from other kinds of optic atrophy. Drusen of the optic disc should not be confused with optic atrophy.

HISTOPATHOLOGICALLY, descending, ascending and post-inflammatory optic atrophy are characterized by degeneration of the nerve fibers, glial proliferation and increase of the collagenous tissue in the pial septa.

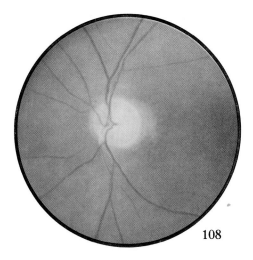

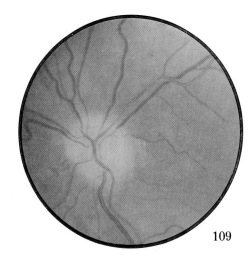

108

109

*Left eye. Vascular optic atrophy. Disc is yellowish-white and slightly cupped.*

*Left eye. Vascular optic atrophy. The disc is pale and slightly cupped.*

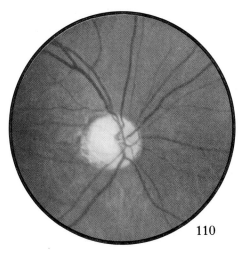

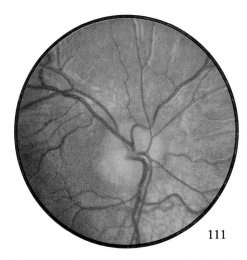

110

111

*Right eye. Optic nerve atrophy in encephalomyelitis. The disc is pale.*

*Right eye. Optic nerve atrophy following chronic papilledema in cranial dysostosis.*

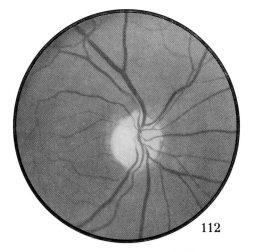

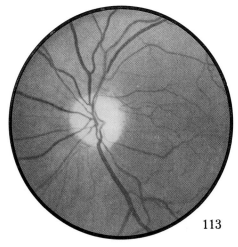

112

113

*Figures 112 and 113. Right and left eyes. Hereditary optic atrophy. Both discs are pale,*

*yellowish-white and slightly cupped. Retinal vessels are normal.*

# Optic Neuritis
(Figures 114—119)

Acute optic neuritis is an inflammatory affection of the optic nerve. If the nerve head or disc is involved, the term papillitis is used. If the lesion lies in the optic nerve behind the lamina cribrosa, the term retrobulbar neuritis is applied.

Optic neuritis may occur in such conditions as intraocular and orbital inflammations, inflammation of the nasal sinuses, in syphilis, diabetes, encephalitis and meningitis. In multiple (disseminated) sclerosis, the neuritis is nearly always retrobulbar. In many cases, however, the cause of neuritis is unknown.

Optic neuritis most often develops in young adults. It is usually unilateral, but may occur bilaterally.

The symptoms usually start quite suddenly with hazy vision, and vision may be reduced to counting of fingers or even light perception. Sometimes, the patient also complains of some retrobulbar pain on movement of or pressure upon the bulb. The visual field shows a central or paracentral scotoma with absolute or relative loss to colors, but rarely sector-formed or peripheral field defects. The blind spot is enlarged.

Neuritis often disappears within a few weeks, leaving no or only slight reduction of vision or defects in the visual fields, although the optic disc may show permanent pallor of the temporal part of the disc or the whole disc.

OPHTHALMOSCOPICALLY, papillitis (Fig. 114) is often indistinguishable from papilledema. Fully developed, however, papillitis may be less strictly limited to the disc, and prepapillary there is often some vitreous haze. The prominence of the swelling of the disc is usually less, and the color of the disc usually more red than in papilledema. Hemorrhages often occur as splinter or flame-shaped hemorrhages on or around the optic disc, and the retinal veins are usually congested. When papillitis subsides, the optic disc may regain its normal appearance. Most often, however, papillitis is followed by a varying degree of pallor of the optic disc (Figs. 115—118).

In the differential diagnosis, papilledema, pseudopapilledema and drusen of the optic disc have to be considered.

In acute retrobulbar neuritis the disc has a normal appearance. Weeks or months later, a sector-formed pallor may develop at the temporal side of the optic disc (Fig. 119).

HISTOPATHOLOGICALLY, papillitis is characterized by edema of the optic nerve head and the adjacent retina, accumulation of inflammatory cells, proliferation of the interstitial tissue and degeneration of the neural tissue, fullness of the veins and sometimes hemorrhages and exudates. Retrobulbar neuritis shows inflammatory and degenerative changes in the optic nerve behind the lamina cribrosa.

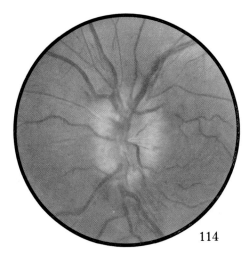

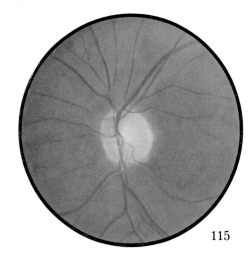

114

115

*Left eye. Optic neuritis. The optic disc is swollen and ill-defined.*

*Same eye as figure 114, eight months later. Postneuritic optic atrophy.*

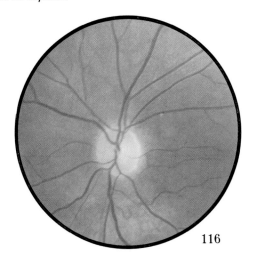

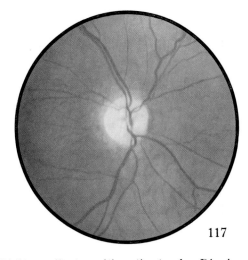

116

117

*Left eye. Postneuritic optic atrophy. The disc is pale and cupped.*

*Right eye. Postneuritic optic atrophy. Disc is pale and slightly cupped.*

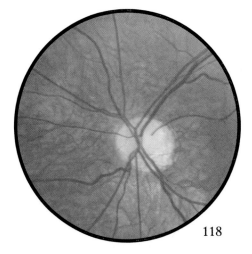

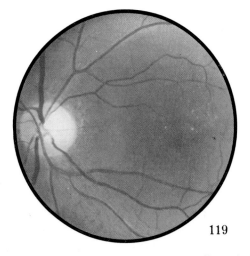

118

119

*Left eye. Postneuritic optic atrophy. The disc is pale and cupped.*

*Left eye. Temporal sectorformed pallor of the disc after retrobulbar neuritis.*

# Glaucomatous Optic Disc Changes
### (Figures 120—125 and 161)

Glaucoma is a condition due to various mechanisms, and characterized by elevation of the intraocular pressure.

Glaucoma may be primary or secondary. Cases of primary glaucoma are usually bilateral and can be divided into closed-angle, chronic simple, juvenile, congenital and absolute glaucoma. The most common form is chronic simple glaucoma. Secondary glaucoma is usually unilateral and a result of inflammatory, vascular, traumatic or neoplastic diseases of the eye.

In all kinds of long-standing ocular hypertension, vision may decrease and characteristic changes develop in the visual field and the optic disc.

The two principal types of glaucoma, closed-angle glaucoma and chronic simple glaucoma which is open-angled, will be discussed in the following.

Closed-angle glaucoma is usually bilateral, although the acute attack often involves one eye only. In the majority of cases, acute closed-angle glaucoma is preceded by prodromal attacks which arise suddenly and subside spontaneously within a few hours. The prodromal attack is similar to the acute attack, but milder. During the acute attack, the intraocular pressure is much increased and colored halos are observed around lights. Vision is blurred and reduced in varying degrees, and may be diminished even to light perception. There is intense pain in the ocular region, radiating into the temporal region. The eyelids may show some edema, there is considerable lacrimation, intense congestion of the bulbar conjunctiva, edema of the cornea—which loses its transparency—and shallow anterior chamber. The pupil is moderately dilated and rigid, and the chamber angle closed.

If normal or approximately normal intraocular tension is re-established within twenty-four to forty-eight hours, useful vision is usually restored. If not, vision is seriously damaged or lost.

OPHTHALMOSCOPIC EXAMINATION is seldom possible during the acute attack. When it is possible, the disc appears somewhat hyperemic (Fig. 124), pulsation may be observed in the central retinal artery and the retinal veins are engorged, but the disc is never pathologically cupped during the first attack.

Chronic simple glaucoma is usually bilateral, but often affects the eyes unequally. It starts insidiously with increased intraocular pressure and progresses very slowly, giving no symptoms until the advanced stage, where characteristic visual defects and reduction in visual acuity develop. The anterior chamber is of normal depth and the chamber angle is open.

OPHTHALMOSCOPICALLY, the early stages of chronic simple glaucoma show no visible fundus changes. In long-standing cases, however, the disc becomes paler and the central retinal vessels are displaced nasally. The pathological cupping

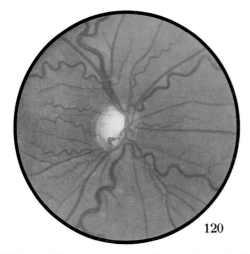

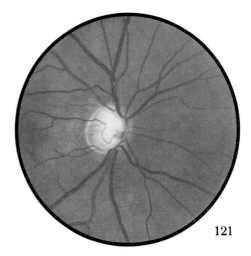

*Right eye. Glaucomatous cupping of the optic disc in buphthalmos.*

*Right eye. Glaucomatous cupping of the optic disc in juvenile glaucoma.*

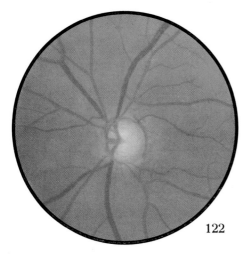

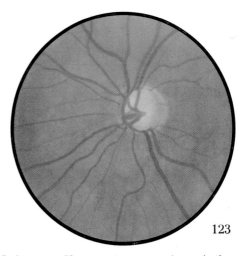

*Left eye. Glaucomatous cupping of the optic disc. The disc is pale, atrophic.*

*Left eye. Glaucomatous cupping of the optic disc. The disc is pale, atrophic.*

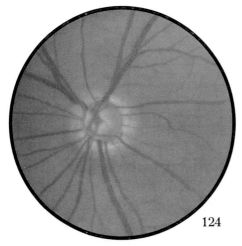

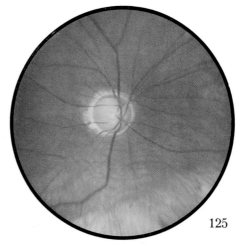

*Left eye. Glaucomatous cupping of the optic disc and acute glaucoma attack.*

*Right eye. Glaucomatous cupping of the optic disc in an aphakic eye.*

of the disc starts temporally (Fig. 120) and proceeds until it occupies the full extent of the disc (Figs. 121—125, 161). Fully developed, the glaucomatous optic disc is atrophic, whitish, yellowish-white or grayish-white and deeply cupped, and the lamina cribrosa, displaced backwards, is seen plainly at the base. At the disc margin the cup shows an abrupt step down from the retinal level. If the margin becomes undermined, the retinal vessels disappear from ophthalmoscopic view when running under the overhanging edge of the cupped disc, and bend sharply as they reappear at the edge. The retinal vessels, therefore, appear as if broken off at the disc margin. Peripapillary, the disc is often surrounded by a whitish or yellowish-white atrophic zone known as glaucomatous halo (Figs. 124—125). The retinal vessels show no characteristic changes.

In the differential diagnosis, other kinds of optic atrophy, senile peripapillary atrophy and pronounced physiological excavation of the disc have to be considered.

HISTOPATHOLOGICALLY, long-standing glaucoma is characterized by backwards displacement of the lamina cribrosa, cupping of the optic disc and cavernous atrophy of the optic nerve. The retina shows degeneration of the nerve fiber, ganglion cell and internal nuclear layers, while the outer retinal layers usually remain normal. Choroidal atrophy occurs, principally in the peripapillary region.

# The Retinal Vessels

## Physiological Variations and Congenital Abnormalities.
### (Figures 1—9, 72—77 and 126—143)

The retinal vessels are usually termed arteries and veins, but from a histological point of view, these vessels are correctly described as arterioles and venules.

The central retinal artery and vein normally appear close to each other at the nasal side of the center of the optic disc (Figs. 1—9). Within the disc margin, they usually divide into a large superior and inferior branch and soon after into a large temporal and nasal branch. Four principal divisions are thereby formed, supplying the four quadrants of the fundus. At the disc, small vessels also leave the main trunks in a temporal and nasal direction. From the disc, the four principal divisions of the retinal vessels take a slightly sinuous course as they proceed into their respective quadrants and divide dichotomously into innumerable

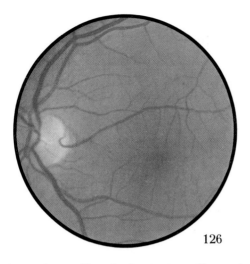

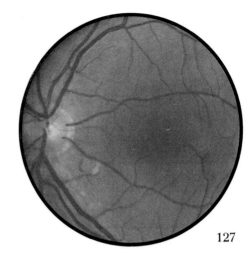

126

127

*Left eye. Large cilioretinal artery supplies part of the macular area.*

*Left eye. Two cilioretinal arteries supply the macular area.*

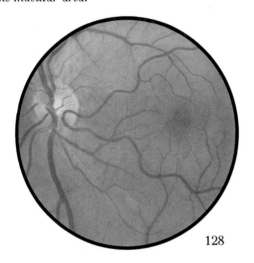

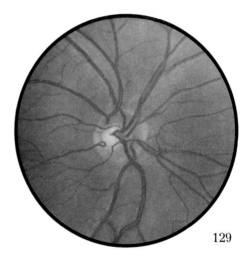

128

129

*Left eye. Two cilioretinal arteries supply the macular area.*

*Right eye. The retinal arteries appear on the disc as three separate trunks.*

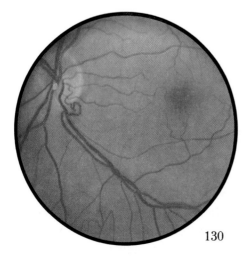

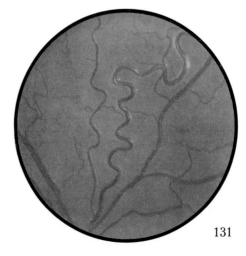

130

131

*Left eye. Abnormal looping and twisting of the lower temporal retinal artery.*

*Right eye. Abnormal tortuosity of retinal vessels in Sturge-Weber's syndrome.*

branches. Passing through the fundus, the retinal arteries and veins cross each other at many points, and as a rule the vein dips below the artery at the crossing. In the periphery, the vascular system stops about one mm behind the ciliary body. In the macular area there is a capillary-free zone of about 0.5 mm corresponding to the fovea centralis.

HISTOLOGICALLY, those parts of the central retinal artery and vein running in the optic nerve are true artery and vein, corresponding to those of comparable size in other situations. After piercing the lamina cribrosa and entering the retina, the arteries soon lose their internal elastic lamina and their multi-layered muscular coat, and in the retina, therefore, are correctly described as arterioles and venules. A single layer of muscle fibers is usually found in the wall of the arteriole, for a considerable part of its way in the retina. In the fundal periphery, however, the arterioles contain no muscle fibers.

The retinal arteries are end-arteries. The arteries appear lighter red and narrower than the dark-red or purplish veins, and normally the arteriovenous ratio is about 2:3. The retinal vessels have a continuous yellow-white light reflex axially. The arterial reflex is more brilliant than the venous, and covers about one third of the arterial and one fourth to one fifth of the venous blood column.

At the disc, pulsation is often found as a physiological condition in the vein, while pulsation in the arteries is only observed in pathological conditions. Arterial pulsation may be observed as locomotion pulse or volume pulse. The first may occur in coarctation of the aorta, and the second in glaucoma, in incom-plete occlusion of the central retinal artery or in aortic insufficiency.

However, the arrangement of the retinal vessels as described is subject to many minor or major physiological variations, and a few will be mentioned below.

A cilioretinal artery (Fig. 126), a branch from the short posterior ciliary arteries, appears separately in about 10 per cent of the cases, usually in the temporal part of the disc, and supplies a smaller or larger part of the macular area. More than one cilioretinal artery may occasionally be present (Figs. 127—128). The cilioretinal arteries may become important in cases of occlusion of the central retinal artery, since the area supplied by the cilioretinal artery is left intact (Fig. 210). On the other hand, occlusion of a cilioretinal artery, which is a rare condition, may damage central vision severely (Fig. 211).

At times, the retinal vessels divide behind the lamina cribrosa and then make their appearance on the disc as two or four branches (Fig. 129). They may also emerge from the upper (Figs. 75—77) or temporal (Figs. 72—74) part of the disc, being accompanied by some deformity of the disc and, respectively, an inferior and nasal crescent.

Occasionally, remnants of the hyaloid artery are seen as a grayish-white cord extending forwards from the optic disc into the vitreous and often ending in a disc-like manner at the posterior lens capsule (Fig. 36).

The retinal vessels may show abnormalities in their course, including vas-

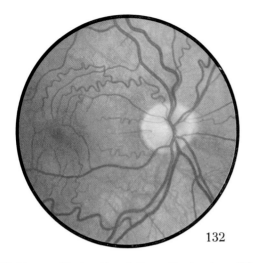

132

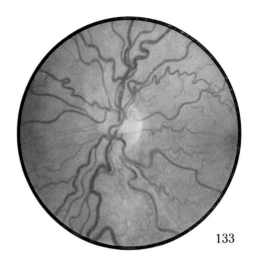

133

*Right eye. Tortuosity of the retinal veins. The retinal arteries are normal.*

*Left eye. Tortuosity of the retinal arteries and veins.*

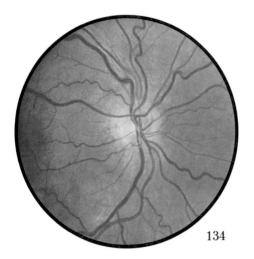

134

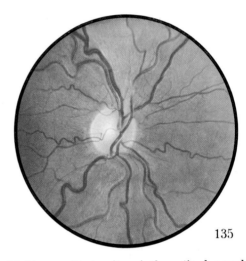

135

*Right eye. Tortuosity of the retinal veins in coarctation of the aorta.*

*Right eye. Tortuosity of the retinal vessels in coarctation of the aorta.*

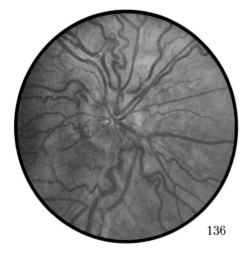

136

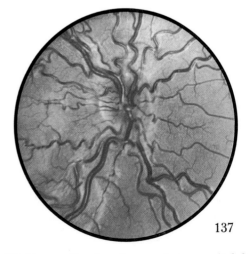

137

*Right eye. Fundus changes in congenital heart disease with cyanosis.*

*Right eye. Fundus changes in congenital heart disease with cyanosis.*

cular tortuousity (Figs. 131—133), and the retinal artery and vein may even be twisted around each other (Fig. 130). The retinal vessels may show abnormal dilatations, abnormal crossings, abnormal directions, abnormal vascular loops and finally abnormal vascular communications.

In congenital tortuousity of the retinal vessels (Figs. 131—133), the arteries or veins, or both arteries and veins appear tortuous and lengthened, but their size and color are normal and the disc is normal.

In coarctation of the aorta (Figs. 134—135), the retinal vessels often show some tortuosity and a locomotion pulse may be present.

In congenital heart disease with cyanosis (Figs. 136—137), the retinal vessels are more or less tortuous and also dilated. The arteries are dark-red or purplish and the veins cyanotic. The disc is reddened and the disc margin often blurred. Fully developed, papilledema may occasionally be present.

Abnormal vascular communications may occur as a simple communication between an artery and a vein (Fig. 138) or between two arteries. In this rare congenital abnormality the retinal vessels often show racemose dilatations. The condition is therefore often referred to as racemose hemangioma or arteriovenous aneurysm of the retina (Fig. 139). This abnormality is often confined to the retina. Sometimes, however, vascular abnormalities may coexist in the orbit and in the midbrain, as in the Wyburn-Mason syndrome. The affected retinal vessels are congested and tortuous, sometimes forming loops or coils in which arteries are difficult or impossible to differentiate from veins. Occasionally, gross dilatation of the retinal vessels may occur without obvious angioma or aneurysm formation. The condition may sometimes be associated with facial and orbital hemangioma (Fig. 140).

Another rare congenital abnormality is retinal cavernous hemangioma which is characterized by telangiectasia of the retinal vessels, resembling miliary aneurysms. Some hemorrhage may also be present. The condition is located in a circumscribed, elevated area with some pigmentation in the fundus periphery, usually in the lower nasal quadrant (Figs. 141—143). The condition may be associated with retinal or preretinal veils of connective tissue.

The lesion gives no visual disturbances unless a hemorrhage develops and bursts into the vitreous. The condition which is usually non-progressive and shows no exudates, must not be confused with early stages of Coats' syndrome or angiomatosis of the retina.

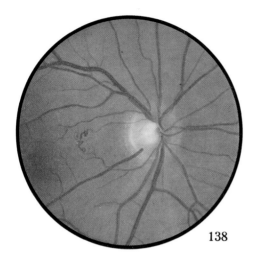

138

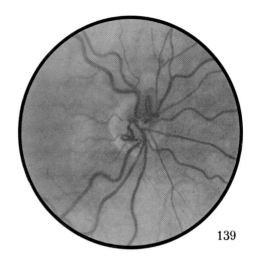

139

*Right eye. Arteriovenous anastomosis with aneurysm formation.*

*Right eye. Racemose hemangioma of the retina at the optic disc.*

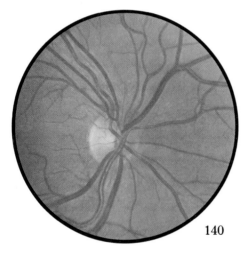

140

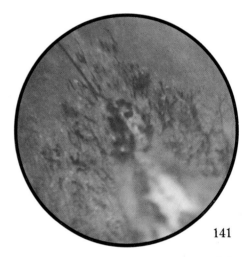

141

*Right eye. Abnormally dilated retinal vessels in orbital hemangioma.*

*Right eye. Congenital cavernous retinal hemangioma.*

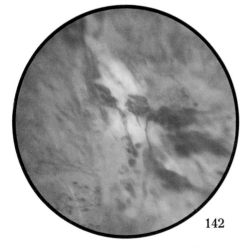

142

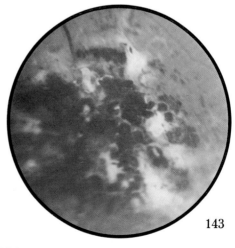

143

*Same eye as figure 141. Congenital cavernous retinal hemangioma.*

*Right eye. Congenital cavernous retinal hemangioma.*

# Angiomatosis of the Retina
(Figures 144—157)

Angiomatosis of the retina is a rare, congenital and frequently familial angioblastic retinal malformation. When confined to the retina it is known as von Hippel's disease. Associated with cerebellar cysts or visceral lesions it is known as von Hippel-Lindau's syndrome.

Angiomatosis may be observed at all ages, but most frequently it is discovered in the twenties or the thirties. The lesion is bilateral in about 50 per cent of the cases.

In early stages vision remains unaltered. Later, however, visual field defects develop in the presence of massive retinal exudates. Gross intraocular hemorrhage may occur at any stage. In the advanced stages the tumor often produces retinal detachment and finally painful secondary glaucoma. In these stages vision is severely impaired.

Angiomatous tumors are frequently situated in the peripheral part of the fundus (Figs. 147, 150—153, 157), but angiomatous tumors may occur at the disc (Figs. 144—145) or even in the macular area. They are usually single but multiple tumors may occur in the same eye.

General symptoms usually start later than the eye symptoms, but may occur even before those symptoms have developed. The most frequent general symptom is evidence of intracranial hemorrhage from an angiomatous tumor in the cerebellum, and such hemorrhages are frequently the cause of the patient's death.

OPHTHALMOSCOPICALLY, the fundus lesion may start in one of two ways. In some cases it commences with enlargement and tortuosity of a major retinal vein, which is soon followed by enlargement of the accompanying artery, but not until later is a retinal tumor visible. In other cases the condition commences as a small vascular tumor in the fundus, followed by enlargement and tortuousity of the vessels supplying the tumor. Characteristically, an angiomatous tumor is supplied by a single dilated and tortuous artery and vein, and it is often difficult to distinguish which is the artery and which is the vein. An angiomatous tumor is seen as a yellowish or whitish (Figs. 144—145, 157) or as a reddish (Figs. 147, 150—153) mass in the retina, measuring from about half a disc diameter to about four disc diameters and projecting forward for a variable distance. In the early stage, there are no or only sparsely scattered exudates (Figs. 150—154), but later, massive whitish or yellowish-white deeply situated exudates develop, at first in the areas neighboring the tumor (Figs. 155—156). Later, the exudate becomes more widespread (Figs. 146—147). Finally, retinal detachment develops (Figs. 148—149). Vitreous hemorrhage is not infrequent and may obscure the ophthalmoscopic picture at any stage.

Angiomatosis of the retina is easy to diagnose in fully developed cases.

In early stages with dilation and tortuosity of retinal vessels but without visi-

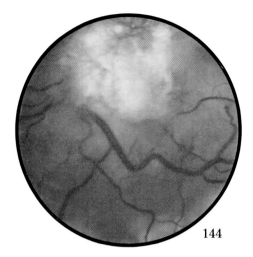

144

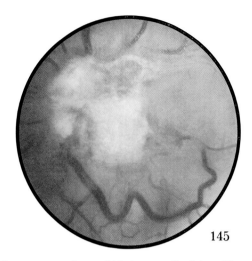

145

*Left eye. Angiomatosis of the retina with prepapillary mass of whitish tissue.*

*Same eye as figure 144, ten months later. Changes have progressed.*

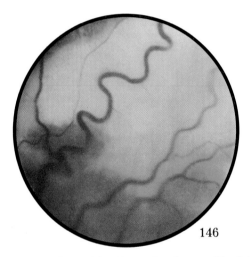

146

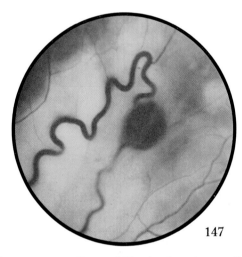

147

*Same eye as figure 145. Extensive dense yellowish retinal and subretinal exudate.*

*Same eye as figure 146. Angiomatous retinal tumor supplied by a single artery and vein.*

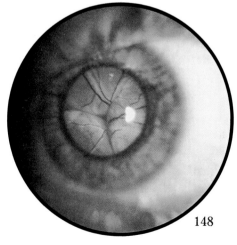

148

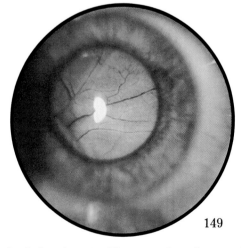

149

*Figures 148 and 149. From the same eye as figures 144—147, nine months later. Total*

*retinal detachment. The extensive, dense yellowish exudate is still present.*

ble angioma, the condition may be confused with racemose hemangioma of the retina or a condition with similar changes in the retina and vascular lesions in the midbrain, the Wyburn-Mason syndrome. Also Coats' syndrome and Eales' disease must be considered in the differential diagnosis. Coats' syndrome is characterized by massive, deep retinal and subretinal exudates and miliary aneurysms, or by miliary aneurysms together with some deeply situated exudate. It is differentiated from angiomatosis of the retina by the lack of angiomatous tumors. Eales' disease is characterized by sheathing of the retinal vessels, new vessel formation and recurrent vitreous hemorrhage. It is differentiated from angiomatosis of the retina by the lack of massive exudate and angiomatous tumor.

HISTOPATHOLOGICALLY, the tumor consists of new-formed capillary vessels and solid cords of endothelial cells, both arising from angioblasts and lying in a cellular matrix with an abundance of glial cells. Secondary changes are often present, such as cystic cavities, gliosis, lipid-laden macrophages and accumulations of exudative material between the choroid and the retina.

# Tuberous Sclerosis
## (Figures 158—159)

Tuberous sclerosis is a rare congenital, heredofamilial disease characterized by adenoma sebaceum, mental deficiency and epilepsy.

Adenoma sebaceum, which may be present from infancy, is characterized by highly vascularized skin papules usually arranged about the nose and cheeks. Mental retardation usually appears during childhood. The disease is usually fatal, the majority of patients dying before the age of 25 years as epileptic idiots, and multiple tuberous tumors may be present in the cerebrum as well as in other organs.

Involvement of the fundus is rare. The fundus lesions may occasionally give rise to visual disturbances and decreased vision.

OPHTHALMOSCOPICALLY, tuberous fundus lesions may appear in two different types. The first type is usually situated pre-papillary and is seen as a large nodular tumor about the size of the optic disc or even larger, and projecting forwards into the vitreous (Fig. 158). The surface of the tumor may be smooth or studded with nodules like a mulberry, and the color of the tumor is grayish-white or yellowish-white. Occasionally, buds may break off from this type of tumor and float freely into the vitreous or settle elsewhere in the retina. The second type of tuberous fundus lesion appears elsewhere in the fundus. It is seen as an oval or round, flat, white or grayish area in the retina, with an average diameter of about half that of the disc or less (Fig. 159).

Multiple tumors, especially of the second type, may be present in the same fundus. Both types of tuberous tumors appear to be relatively avascular, and the lesions are only slightly progressive.

Conditions that must be considered in the differential diagnosis are angiomatosis of the retina with papillary localization, and neurofibromatosis. The tuberous lesion is differentiated ophthalmoscopically from angiomatosis of the retina by the avascularity of the tuberous tumor

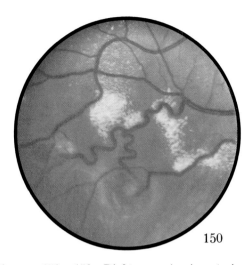

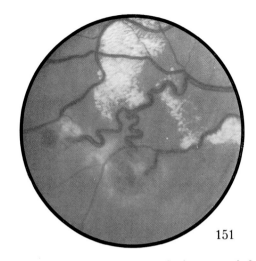

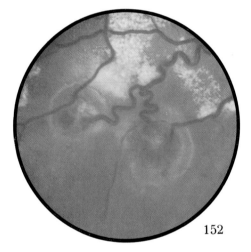

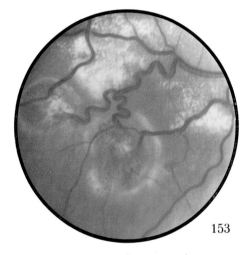

*Figures 150—153. Right eye. Angiomatosis of the retina. The pictures show the development of two angiomatous tumors during a period of one year. Both tumors are supplied by a single*

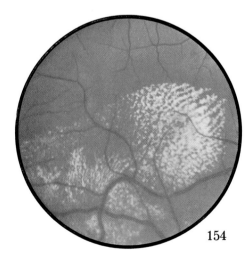

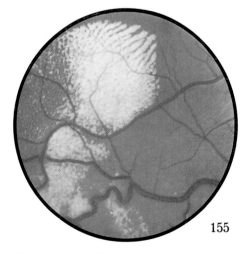

*artery and vein. Yellowish retinal exudate formation shows a steady progression.*

*Figures 154 and 155. Same eye as figures 150—153. Progressive formation of dense yellowish-white exudate during a period of about one year.*

and the lack of exudates. Furthermore the conditions are distinguished by differences in the general clinical appearance. In neurofibromatosis the fundus lesion may be very similar to that in tuberous sclerosis, and the conditions must therefore be separated by the general signs.

HISTOPATHOLOGICALLY, the tumors are composed of polymorphic fibrous astrocytes with an oval nucleus and indistinct cell boundaries. The tumors usually lie superficially and do not destroy the internal limiting membrane or infiltrate retinal structures other than the nerve fiber or the ganglion cell layers.

# Sturge-Weber's Syndrome
### (Figures 120 and 160—161)

Sturge-Weber's syndrome consists of a triad of symptoms: facial capillary angioma, intracranial angioma, and choroidal angioma with or without buphthalmos. All symptoms may not be present at the same time. Incomplete forms are more frequent than the complete syndrome.

The cutaneous capillary angioma, nevus flammeus, may be present at birth. It is usually unilateral and limited to the distribution of the first and second divisions of the trigeminal nerve.

Intracranial angiomas in the pia are usually situated on the same side as the nevus flammeus and are later associated with progressive calcification within the underlying cerebral cortex. Sooner or later a variable degree of cerebral atrophy develops, and this atrophy is followed by progressive mental deterioration and epileptiform attacks.

Choroidal angiomas may give rise to raised intraocular tension with or without buphthalmos. Visual disturbances and visual field defects may subsequently occur as a result of the raised intraocular tension.

OPHTHALMOSCOPICALLY, choroidal angiomas are seen as localized (Fig. 161) or more diffuse (Fig. 160) yellowish or yellowish-gray flat areas anywhere in the fundus. The retinal vessels may be tortuous and somewhat dilated (Fig. 120) and sometimes show a bizarre configuration (Fig. 160).

In cases with long-standing glaucoma, glaucomatous optic disc changes may occur in the form of atrophy and cupping of the optic nerve head (Figs. 120 and 161).

In the differential diagnosis, malignant choroidal melanoma must be considered. The two conditions can sometimes be distinguished by fluorescein angiography, as choroidal angiomas may show a fluorescein pattern, differing from that seen in malignant choroidal melanoma.

HISTOPATHOLOGICALLY, choroidal angiomas consist of endothelial-lined spaces of varying sizes, engorged with blood and separated by scanty connective tissue stroma. Over the tumor the retina may show degenerative changes in the form of microcyst formation. The optic disc may show glaucomatous cupping and atrophy, and there may be cavernous atrophy of the optic nerve.

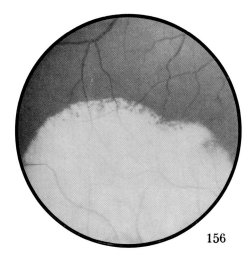

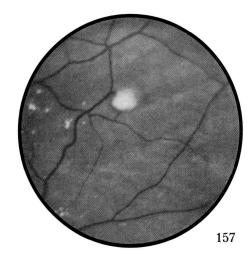

156

157

*Same eye as figure 155, three years later. The exudate has increased in size.*

*Right eye. Angiomatous tumor in the upper nasal quadrant of the eye.*

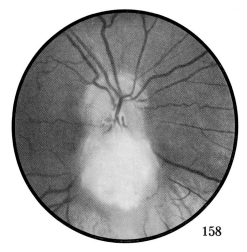

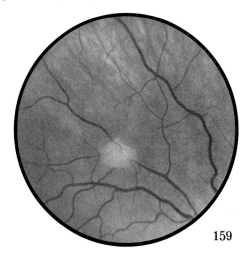

158

159

*Right eye. Tuberous sclerosis. Yellowish-white tumor below the disc.*

*Same eye as figure 158. Grayish-white nodule in the upper temporal quadrant.*

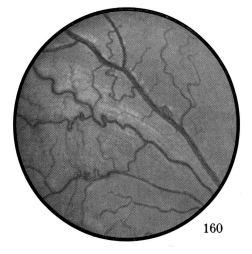

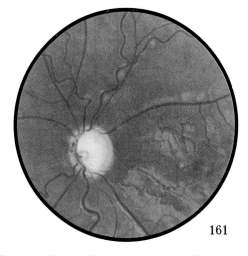

160

161

*Right eye. Sturge-Weber's syndrome. Ill-defined yellowish-orange choroidal angioma.*

*Left eye. Sturge-Weber's syndrome. Glaucomatous disc and choroidal angiomas.*

# Sclerosis of the Retinal Vessels

(Figures 162—167, 180—181, 209, 218—220, 238—239 and 252—253)

As the retinal vessels are visible ophthalmoscopically, the development of retinal vascular sclerosis can readily be followed in the fundus.

Retinal vascular sclerosis is indicated by some of the following lesions: changes in the arterial light reflex, arteriovenous crossing phenomena, variations in caliber or course, or sheathing of the retinal vessels.

Involuntary sclerosis of the retinal vessels is an almost physiological process related to aging, normally found in healthy persons in the sixties and later. The condition is seldom present before the age of 50 years, and never in the young. The fundus changes consist of some narrowing and slight variations in caliber of the retinal arteries, broadening of the arterial light reflex (copper-wire arteries) and slight or moderate arteriovenous crossing phenomena.

More advanced retinal vascular sclerosis occurs in cases of involuntary sclerosis associated with hypertension, and in cases of long-standing hypertension and long-standing diabetes where the disease itself produces or accelerates the development of retinal vascular sclerosis. Advanced vascular sclerosis is characterized by moderate narrowing and some variation in caliber of the retinal arteries, copper- or silver-wire arteries, moderate or pronounced crossing phenomena and sometimes, atheromatous plaques or sheathing of the retinal vessels.

Involuntary retinal vascular sclerosis as a rule does not affect the visual acuity.

In advanced vascular sclerosis, however, degenerative retinal changes may induce visual disturbances.

OPHTHALMOSCOPICALLY, in involuntary or moderate sclerosis, the retinal arteries are slightly narrowed and the axial arterial light reflex is less bright, more diffuse and broader than normal (Figs. 162, 164—165), giving the artery the appearance of a copper-wire (copper-wire arteries). In advanced sclerosis, the arteries are narrow and the axial reflex is broad, very pale and whitish (Figs. 180—181), giving the artery the appearance of a silver-wire (silver-wire arteries).

Arteriovenous crossing phenomena may occur as Gunn's sign or Salus' sign. Gunn's sign is seen as a pale zone of the vein or a concealment of the vein on both sides of the crossing artery (Figs. 163—167). The width of this pale zone varies. In involuntary or moderate sclerosis, the pale zone of the vein is always small or only slightly indicated, while in advanced sclerosis the vein may show tapered ends or terminate abruptly at some distance from the artery, leaving a pale zone on each side of the artery (Figs. 180—181). At the arteriovenous crossing, the artery and the vein have a common adventitial coat and the apparent narrowing or concealment of the vein is due to a gradual loss of transparency in the arterial wall and the perivascular tissue.

At times, the vein shows some twisting and distension peripheral to the crossing, centrally it is straighter and narrower for a short distance and then resumes

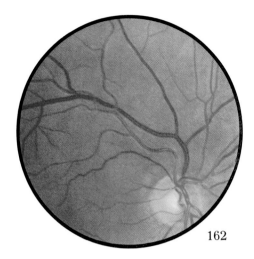

162

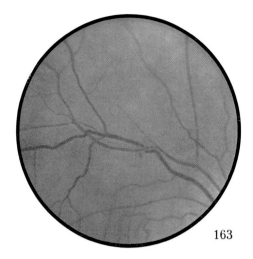

163

*Right eye. Slight sclerosis of the retinal vessels (copper-wire arteries).*

*Right eye. Moderate sclerosis with typical arteriovenous crossing phenomena.*

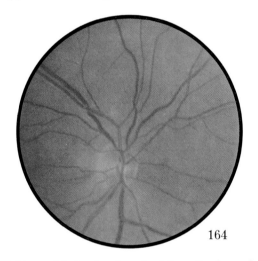

164

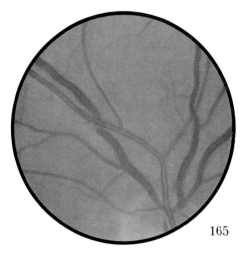

165

*Right eye. Moderate sclerosis of the retinal vessels.*

*Same eye as figure 164 (15°). Arteriovenous crossing phenomenon.*

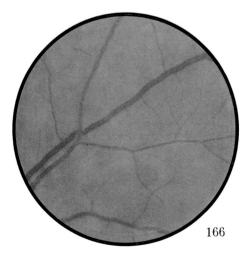

166

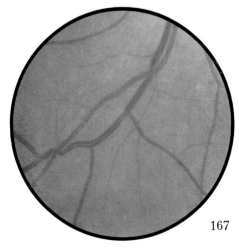

167

*Left eye (15°). Arteriovenous crossing phenomenon.*

*Right eye (15°). Arteriovenous crossing phenomena.*

its normal appearance, a phenomenon known as "banking" (Figs. 163, 166). Salus' sign is seen as an S-formed bend or a U-formed displacement or deflection of the vein which crosses under the artery at right angles instead of obliquely, and associated with some pallor or concealment of the vein on both sides of the crossing artery (Fig. 167).

The sclerosed retinal arteries usually have a straighter course than normal (Fig. 164), branch more acutely, and show some variations in caliber. The retinal veins show slight irregular tortuosities and more or less irregular variations in caliber.

Sheathing of the retinal vessels is due to loss of transparency of the vessel wall. Slight sheathing is often not observed in ordinary ophthalmoscopy, but may readily be seen in red-free light ophthalmoscopy. Advanced sheathing is seen in ordinary ophthalmoscopy as pale, whitish parallel lines along the borders of the blood column (parallel sheathing) (Figs. 209, 220, 252). If sheathing progresses, the blood column may be completely hidden, so that a shorter or longer part of the vessel appears as a solid white strand (pipe-stem sheathing) (Figs. 219, 238—239, 253). Atheromatous plaques may also obscure an artery for a short distance (Fig. 218). Sheathing seems to be due to changes either in the perivascular adventitial sheaths or in the subendothelial tissue. The condition is not only related to the aging process, atheromatous disease or hypertension, but several factors may be concerned and therefore the etiology is still a matter of discussion.

In advanced vascular sclerosis, fundus changes may be present in the form of patchy retinal atrophies, small superficial and deep retinal hemorrhages and small glistening, well-defined white or yellowish-white exudates in the posterior part of the fundus.

Senile macular degeneration and vascular atrophy of the optic disc are discussed elsewhere.

HISTOPATHOLOGICALLY, the retinal vessels present varying degrees of arteriolosclerosis and phlebosclerosis. Fully developed, the sclerosed vessels show localized or generalized thickening, hyalinization and fibrosis of their walls and narrowing of their lumen. Occasionally, atheromatous lesions may be present in the larger retinal vessels. Hemorrhages are superficial and deep. The exudates are deeply situated and composed of albuminous and hyaline material.

# Fundus Changes in Hypertension
### (Figures 96 and 168—197)

The basic fundus lesion in hypertension is an angiospasm, seen as a generalized or localized narrowing of the retinal arteries. If, however, the hypertension is preceded by involuntary sclerosis of the retinal vessels, this angiospasm is more or less obscured by the sclerotic changes.

Hypertensive fundus changes may be classified into retinal angiopathy, retinopathy and neuroretinopathy, and in dis-

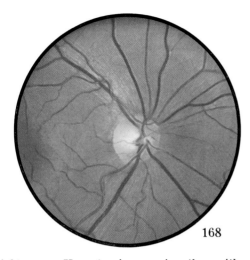

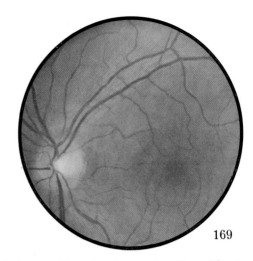

168

169

*Right eye. Hypertensive angiopathy without vascular sclerosis.*

*Left eye. Hypertensive angiopathy without vascular sclerosis.*

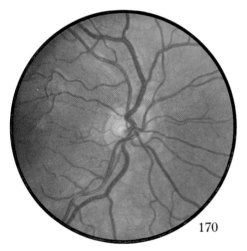

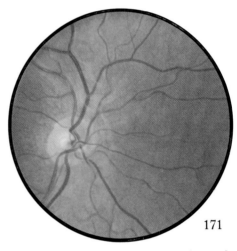

170

171

*Right eye. Normal retinal vessels during anti-hypertensive treatment.*

*Same eye as figure 170, two years later, during exacerbation of hypertension.*

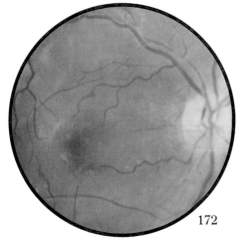

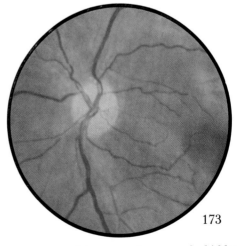

172

173

*Figures 172 and 173. Right and left eyes. Hypertensive angiopathy. The retinal arteries are*

*very narrow and in some places nearly hidden by retinal edema.*

cussing these changes the various forms of hypertension must be distinguished, as the fundus changes and their course vary according to the different conditions.

Moderate chronic hypertension as observed in essential hypertension, some chronic renal, vascular and endocrine disorders etc., may be present for years without any visible fundus changes or may only present a slight narrowing of the retinal arteries. If hypertension persists, retinal angiopathy develops and this angiopathy is mainly seen as an accelerated sclerosis of the retinal vessels. In periods of exacerbation, however, the fundus picture may be altered by the occurrence of hypertensive retinopathy, while neuroretinopathy seldom develops.

Hypertensive fundus changes occurring in acute glumerulonephritis, eclampsia or pre-eclampsia of pregnancy, pheochromocytoma etc., are characterized in the early stages by retinal angiopathy, which is seen as generalized or localized narrowing of the retinal arteries. If blood pressure is not normalized within a short time, the fundus changes progress and retinopathy or even neuroretinopathy develops. The fundus picture, however, usually alters in accordance with remission and exacerbation of the hypertension. If hypertension has been present for a long time, secondary sclerosis invariably develops in the retinal vessels. However, if normal blood pressure is reestablished within a short time, the fundus changes may disappear entirely.

Keith, Wagener and Barker classified the hypertensive fundus changes into four grades according to the prognosis for life. Grade 1 was characterized by mild narrowing or sclerosis of the retinal arteries; grade 2 by generalized or localized irregular narrowing, moderate or marked sclerosis of the retinal arteries and arteriovenous crossing phenomena; grade 3 by the aforementioned vascular changes and retinal edema, cotton-wool exudates and retinal hemorrhages; grade

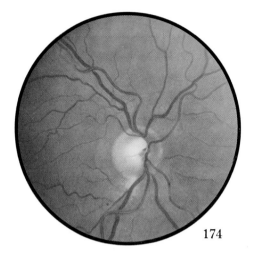

174

*Right eye. Hypertensive angiopathy with vascular sclerosis.*

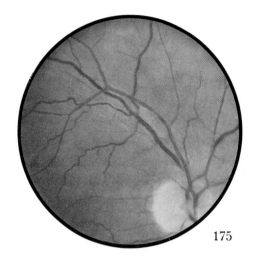

175

*Right eye. Hypertensive angiopathy with vascular sclerosis.*

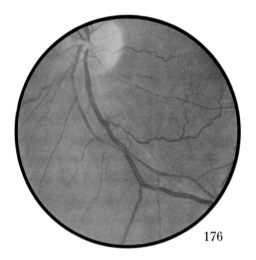

176

*Left eye. Hypertensive angiopathy with vascular sclerosis.*

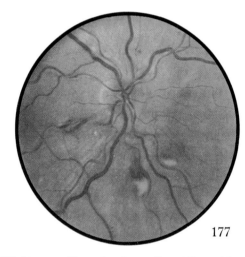

177

*Right eye. Hypertensive retinopathy with hemorrhages and cotton-wool exudates.*

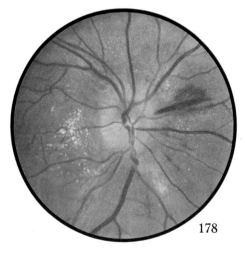

178

*Right eye. Hypertensive retinopathy with hemorrhages and hard exudates.*

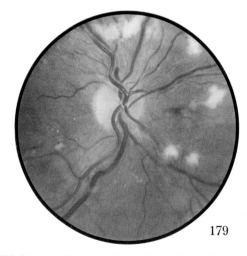

179

*Right eye. Hypertensive retinopathy with cotton-wool exudates and hemorrhage.*

4 by papilledema in addition to the changes found in grade 3.

As the fundus picture usually alters in accordance with the hypertensive state, the ophthalmoscopic examination is of great value for the clinician. The retinal vascular changes, however, are not always in step with the vascular changes in kidney, heart and brain, so that an evaluation of the general prognosis must include evidence of changes in all vascular areas, severity and duration of hypertension, the age of the patient and the response to treatment.

Vision is not altered in hypertensive angiopathy. In hypertensive retinopathy central vision may be reduced if the macula is involved. In hypertensive neuro-retinopathy, vision is usually decreased although the degree of visual reduction may vary considerably.

OPHTHALMOSCOPICALLY, hypertensive angiopathy without vascular sclerosis (Figs. 168—173) is characterized by generalized or localized narrowing of the retinal arteries. In long-standing hypertension or involuntary vascular sclerosis associated with hypertension, however, arteriovenous crossing phenomena and signs of vascular sclerosis are also present (Figs. 174—176). At times, the hypertensive angiopathy is associated with retinal edema (Figs. 172—173). This occurs most frequently in eclampsia or pre-eclampsia of pregnancy, and in cases with acute exacerbation of hypertension.

Hypertensive retinopathy (Figs. 177—184) is characterized by the addition of retinal hemorrhages and exudates and some retinal edema. The hemorrhages consist of superficial, flame-shaped and deep, rounded hemorrhages. The exudates consist of grayish-white or whitish cotton-wool patches, discrete or confluent yellowish-white exudates, and sometimes a macular star, composed of whitish exudates radiating in all directions from the fovea. Slight retinal edema is indicated by an increase in the fundal reflexes, while moderate edema gives the retina a

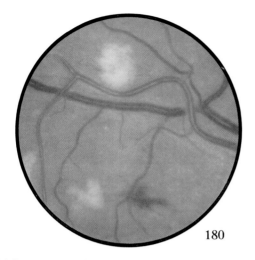

180

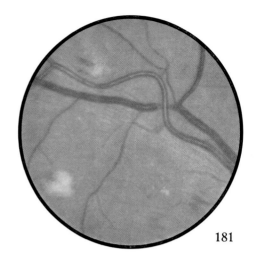

181

*Right eye (15°). Hypertensive retinopathy. Arteriovenous crossing phenomenon.*

*Same eye as figure 180 (15°), two months later. Cotton-wool exudates diminished.*

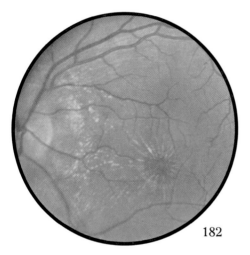

182

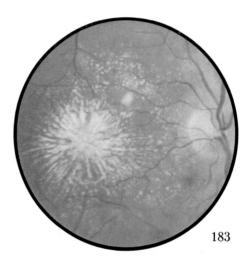

183

*Left eye. Slight macular star formation in hypertensive retinopathy.*

*Right eye. Pronounced macular star formation in hypertensive retinopathy.*

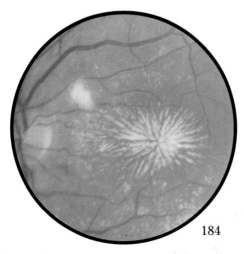

184

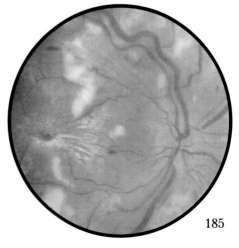

185

*Left eye. Pronounced macular star formation in hypertensive retinopathy.*

*Right eye. Hypertensive neuroretinopathy. The optic disc is edematous.*

more grayish color. In eclampsia, edema may even cause a reversible serous retinal detachment.

Retinal hemorrhages and cotton-wool exudates are often absorbed in the course of some weeks or a few months, leaving no ophthalmoscopic trace, but as new hemorrhages and exudates may develop simultaneously, the general ophthalmoscopic picture is often maintained.

Hypertensive neuroretinopathy (Figs. 96, 185—188, 192) is characterized by the addition of papilledema.

Hypertensive neuroretinopathy should not be confused with occlusion of the central retinal vein or papilledema.

If normal blood pressure is re-established within a short time, retinal edema subsides quickly, and papilledema, retinal hemorrhages and woolly exudates disappear in the course of some weeks or a few months, while hard yellowish-white exudates and a macular star subside very slowly over a period of months (Figs. 192—197), and discrete exudates may persist even for years (Fig. 190). The disappearance of a macular star is often followed by depigmentation and pigment clumping in the macular area (Figs. 196—197), and not infrequently by some persistent reduction of the visual acuity. Retinal hemorrhages and woolly exudates usually disappear leaving no ophthalmoscopic traces, but occasionally visible patchy retinal atrophy develops (Fig. 191). If hypertension has been present for a long time, retinal vascular sclerosis persists even if the blood pressure is normalized (Fig. 189).

HISTOPATHOLOGICALLY, in early stages of hypertension, the ophthalmoscopically visible generalized and localized narrowing of the retinal arteries cannot be demonstrated. In long-standing hypertension, however, the retinal arteries show arteriolosclerosis with medial proliferation and hyalinization, localized adventitial proliferation and fibrosis, and narrowing of the lumen. Flame-shaped hemorrhages are formed in the superficial

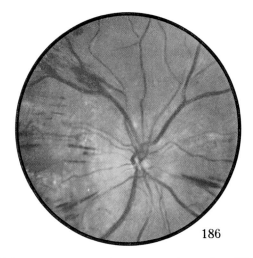

186

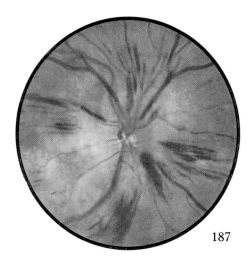

187

*Right eye. Hypertensive neuroretinopathy. The optic disc is swollen.*

*Same eye as figure 186, three weeks later. Fundus changes have progressed.*

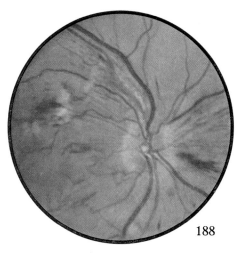

188

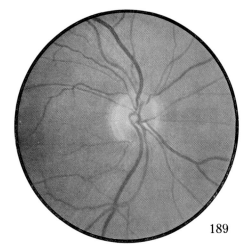

189

*Right eye. Hypertensive neuroretinopathy. The disc is swollen.*

*Same eye as figure 188, seventeen months later. Papilledema has subsided.*

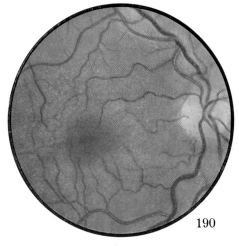

190

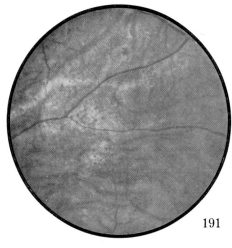

191

*Right eye. Hard exudates as sequelae after hypertensive retinopathy.*

*Right eye. Retinal atrophy after advanced hypertensive retinopathy.*

retinal layers and rounded hemorrhages in the deep layers. The retinal edema involves all layers. The discrete, yellowish-white exudates are found in spaces in the nuclear layers and consist of lipoid, albuminous and fibrinous material. Cotton-wool exudates are localized to the nerve fiber layer, which is swollen and includes the cytoid bodies. These are cell-like bodies possibly representing degenerative changes in the nerve fibers. The cotton-wool exudates probably represent minute ischemic infarcts. A macular star is situated in the outer plexiform layer and is formed by large, fat-filled microglia cells, interspersed by free masses of lipoid and by patches of hyalinized cellular debris.

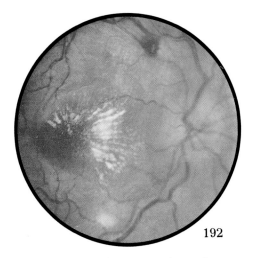

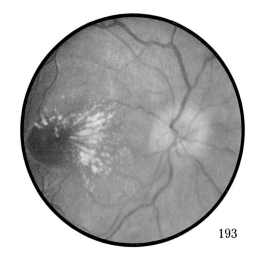

*Right eye. Hypertensive neuroretinopathy.*

*Same eye as figure 192, three weeks later. Retinal edema is in regression.*

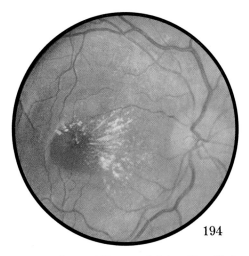

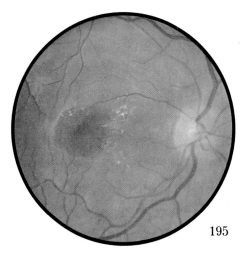

*Same eye as figure 193, a week later. Papilledema in regression.*

*Same eye as figure 194, four months later. Small remnants of macular star.*

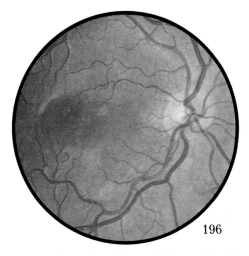

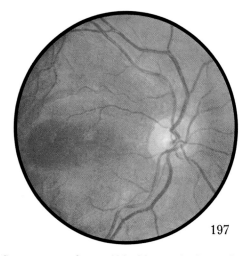

*Same eye as figure 195, 13 months later. Hypertensive changes nearly disappeared.*

*Same eye as figure 196, 28 months later, during exacerbation of hypertension.*

# Occlusion of the Central Retinal Artery and Its Branches

### (Figures 198—221)

Occlusion of the central retinal artery or one of its branches may be the result of thrombotic closure of the lumen, blockage by an embolus or local vasomotor constriction of the vessels. Obstruction by thrombosis due to atheromatous disease with or without hypertension is by far the most common cause of obstruction of the retinal arterial blood flow. An occlusion by a proliferative endarteritis and terminal thrombosis may, however, occur in conditions such as giant-cell arteritis. Blockage of the arterial flow by an embolus is relatively rare. It may occur in conditions such as carotid insufficiency or carotid occlusion, rheumatic heart disease, in auricular fibrillation, and blood diseases such as polycythemia and paraproteinemia. Infective emboli may arise in subacute bacterial endocarditis and other infective illnesses. Fat emboli may occur after injury and air emboli have been recorded following carotid angiography. Blockage of the arterial blood flow by local vasomotor constrictions may also be of some importance.

Occlusion of the central retinal artery occurs most often in middle-aged or elderly persons. The occlusion is usually unilateral but may occur bilaterally.

In some cases, the occlusion is preceded by prodromal obscurations of vision for a variable period before the final attack. At the actual onset of the occlu-

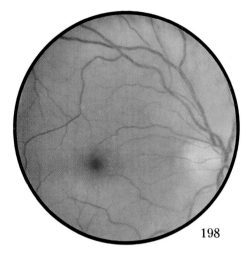

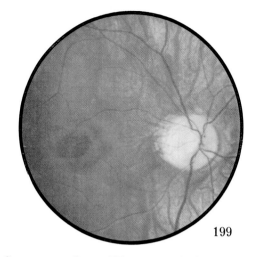

*Right eye. Occlusion of the central retinal artery, acute stage.*

*Same eye as figure 198, two months later. Retinal edema diminished, disc pale.*

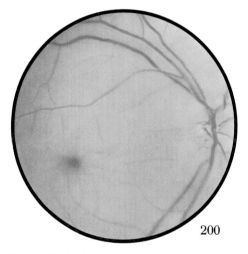

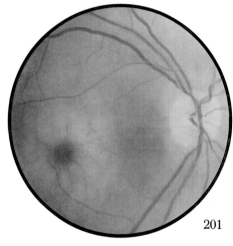

*Right eye. Occlusion of the central retinal artery, acute stage.*

*Same eye as figure 200, ten days later. The retinal edema is in regression.*

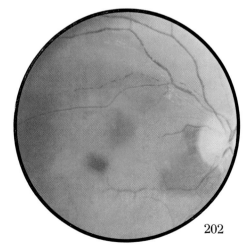

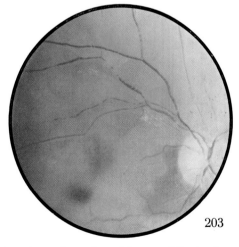

*Figures 202 and 203. Right eye. Occlusion of central retinal artery, acute stage. Fundus is*

*edematous, fovea is red-brown. Blood column is broken up into segments.*

sion of the central retinal artery, the patient suddenly or within a few minutes experiences complete loss of vision in the affected eye, and the pupil becomes wide and does not react to direct light stimulation. If a branch of the central retinal artery is occluded, the visual defect is partial, corresponding to the area supplied by the involved branch. If the obstruction of the blood flow is total for more than one hour, the retina which was supplied by the occluded artery cannot survive and its function is lost. If the obstruction of the blood flow is incomplete or restored within an hour or so, recovery of vision may occur, but most frequently the improvement is incomplete and the eye often becomes blind.

Secondary glaucoma may follow an occlusion of the central retinal artery, usually one or two months after the vascular accident, but secondary glaucoma in this condition is rare compared to the frequency at which it occurs after central venous occlusion.

In rare cases, the clinical picture is altered by the presence of a cilioretinal artery, a branch from the short posterior ciliary arteries. In these cases the area supplied by the cilioretinal artery is normal and the corresponding visual field is spared.

In occlusion of a cilioretinal artery, however, the macular area is involved. Central vision may be completely lost and a centrocoecal scotoma is present, while the rest of the visual field is spared.

OPHTHALMOSCOPICALLY, shortly after the occlusion of the central artery, the retinal arteries are seen as thin or even thread-like, more or less red lines of varying caliber. Sometimes the blood column is broken up into segments which may exhibit slight to-and-fro movements (Figs. 202—203). The arterial light reflexes are narrowed or absent, and arterial pulsation cannot be produced if the occlusion is complete. After a period of narrowing, the arteries may widen again (Figs. 198, 200, 204, 205), but pulsation

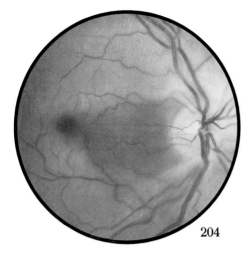

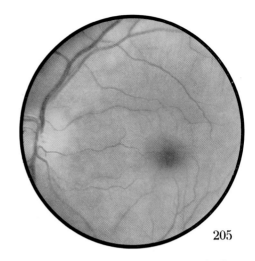

*Right eye. Occlusion of the central retinal artery, acute stage. Cilioretinal artery patent.*

*Left eye. Occlusion of the central retinal artery, acute stage.*

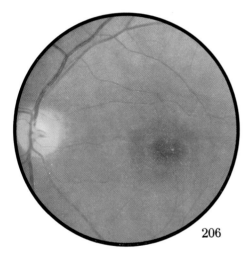

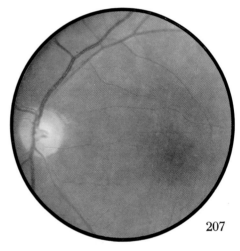

*Same eye as figure 205, three weeks later. Central edema nearly disappeared.*

*Same eye as figure 206, two months later. Slight macular degeneration.*

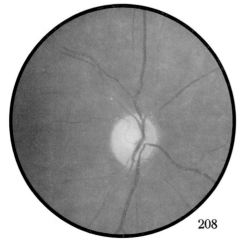

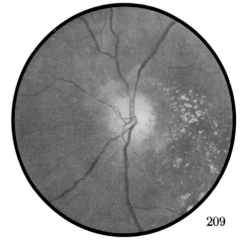

*Right eye. Occlusion of central retinal artery, late stage. Retinal arteries narrow.*

*Left eye. Occlusion of the central retinal artery, late stage.*

still cannot be produced. Within a few hours after the occlusion, the retina becomes pale, opaque, grayish-white or milky, due to edema of the internal retinal layers, and particularly to a cloudy swelling of the ganglion cell layer (Figs. 198, 200, 202, 205). At the fovea, ganglion cells are lacking and the retina is thin. The fovea therefore retains its normal color and appears as a red-brown or cherry-red, rounded spot, contrasting markedly with the surrounding pale retina. The disc is pale and the disc margin indistinct. Retinal hemorrhages are usually absent, but if present they are few in number.

In cases which present a cilioretinal artery (Figs. 204, 210), the area supplied by this vessel is normal and contrasts markedly with the adjacent opaque retina.

In occlusion of a retinal arterial branch (Figs. 212, 214) or occlusion of a cilioretinal artery, the retinal pallor is confined to the area supplied by the occluded branch. In arterial branch occlusion, an embolus or an atheromatous plaque may be present and clearly visible at the site of the occlusion which is usually at a bifurcation of the artery (Figs. 214, 218).

After some time, a certain blood flow is usually re-established, and after some weeks or a few months the retinal edema gradually disappears (Figs. 198—201, 205—207, 212—215). Thereafter, the area involved may gradually assume a more or less granular, atrophic appearance (Fig. 211), often showing pigmentation and glistening, white exudates (Fig. 209). The retinal vessels become narrow and may show more or less pronounced sheathing (Figs. 208—209, 219—220), and in branch occlusion a certain collateral circulation may be established (Figs. 216—217, 221). In the late stage of central retinal artery occlusion, the optic disc becomes pale and atrophic (Figs. 199, 207—209).

The alterations in the retinal blood circulation can readily be followed by fluo-

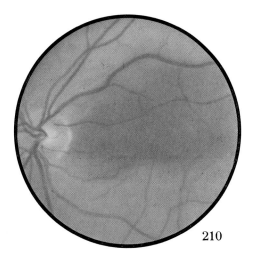

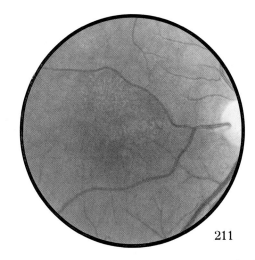

210

211

*Left eye. Occlusion of central retinal artery. Cilioretinal artery patent.*

*Right eye. Macular degeneration after occlusion of cilioretinal artery.*

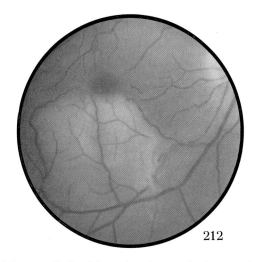

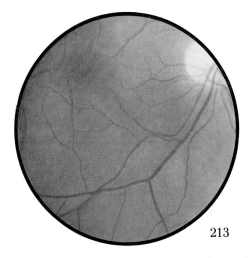

212

213

*Right eye. Retinal branch artery occlusion, acute stage.*

*Same eye as figure 212, six months later. The retinal edema has subsided.*

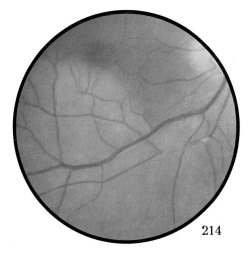

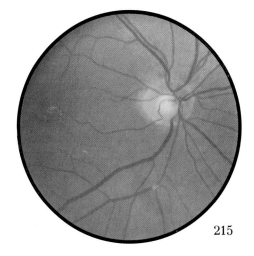

214

215

*Right eye. Retinal branch artery occlusion, acute stage.*

*Same eye as figure 214, five months later. The retinal edema has disappeared.*

rescein angiography.

The ophthalmoscopic picture of central retinal artery occlusion is very characteristic and should not be confused with the ophthalmoscopic picture in Tay-Sachs' disease and Niemann-Pick's disease, which may appear very similar, although the pathogenesis is quite different. Furthermore, occlusion of the central retinal artery usually occurs in middle-aged or elderly persons, while the latter diseases occur only in infancy.

HISTOPATHOLOGICALLY, the central retinal artery may be occluded by a thrombus situated at or just behind the lamina cribrosa, but serial sections are often necessary to reveal the thrombus or its sequelae. The condition is often accompanied by phlebosclerosis of the central retinal vein.

In the early stages, there is marked swelling of the ganglion cells, marked edema and necrosis of the inner two thirds of the retina. Later, this part of the retina becomes totally atrophic, while the outer layers remain normal.

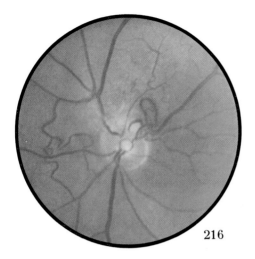

216

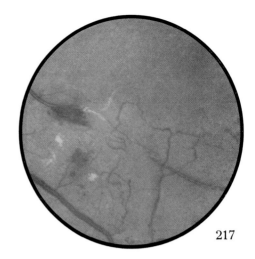

217

*Left eye. Old occlusion of two branches of the central retinal artery.*

*Left eye (15°). Old occlusion of a retinal artery.*

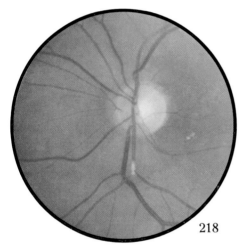

218

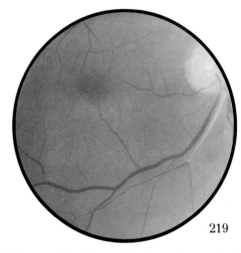

219

*Left eye. Atheromatous plaque at the bifurcation of the lower retinal artery.*

*Right eye. Sheathing of the lower temporal retinal artery.*

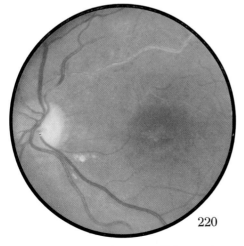

220

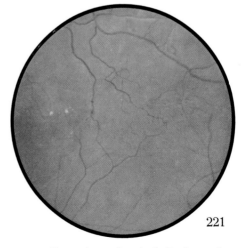

221

*Figures 220 and 221. Left eye. Old branch artery occlusion. Upper temporal artery occluded and*

*corresponding vein ensheathed. Perimacular anastomoses developed.*

# Occlusion of the Central Retinal Vein and Its Branches

(Figures 222—239)

Obstruction of the central retinal vein or a branch of the central retinal vein is a result of a thrombus formation or occlusion of the lumen by proliferated endothelium and subendothelial connective tissue. Several factors may contribute to the obstruction. The most important factor is a sclerotic process involving the central vein as well as the central artery in the posterior part of the lamina cribrosa. A second important factor is stagnation of the circulation caused by the sclerotic process or by impairment of the arterial flow to the eye, or failure of the circulation, as seen in different conditions. Finally, degenerative and inflammatory processes in the veins, as well as primary simple glaucoma, may be factors in the pathogenesis.

In carotid insufficiency or carotid occlusion, cotton-wool exudates, small retinal hemorrhages and microaneurysms may occur without signs of true occlusion of the central retinal vein.

In occlusion of the central retinal vein and its branches, the retinal blood circulation is not completely blocked, but the blood flow is reduced. In the course of some months the circulation becomes more or less re-established by recanalization or the formation of a collateral circulation.

The condition occurs most frequently in elderly persons who exhibit signs of sclerosis of the retinal vessels and often hypertension, but it may also occur in long-standing diabetes, carotid insufficiency or carotid occlusion, polycythemia and other conditions with increased viscosity of the blood such as paraproteinemias, in simple chronic glaucoma, or it may complicate an acute orbitofacial inflammation. The occlusion is usually unilateral, but may also occur bilaterally.

Patients presenting obstruction of the central retinal vein often claim transient obscurations of vision lasting from a few minutes to some hours, some time before the actual onset of the venous blockage. When this occurs, vision becomes impaired within a few hours or characteristically the patients wake up in the morning with impaired vision. Although the vision is often reduced to counting of fingers or hand movements, light perception always remains.

Vision may improve in the course of some months, but as permanent macular damage is common, central vision may remain decreased or even be lost. In about 15 to 20 per cent of the cases, secondary (hemorrhagic) glaucoma develops about two or three months after the onset of the occlusion. In these cases the

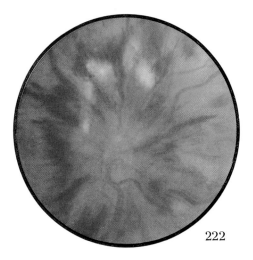

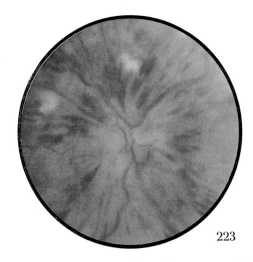

Figures 222 and 223. Right and left eyes. Bilateral occlusion of the central retinal vein, acute stage. The swollen disc surrounded by hemorrhages and cotton-wool exudates.

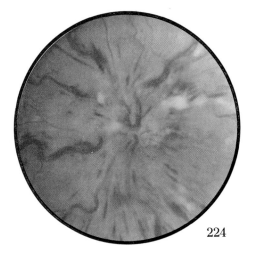

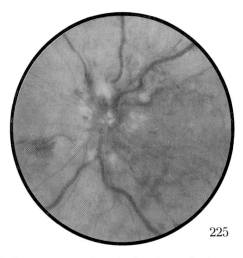

Left eye. Occlusion of the central retinal vein, acute stage.

Left eye. Central retinal vein occlusion, acute stage.

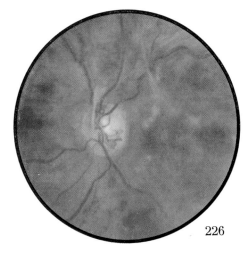

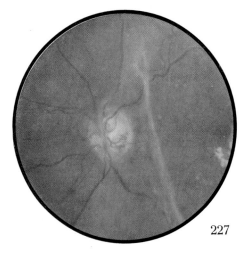

Figures 226 and 227. Same eye as figure 225, four months and six years later. Neovascularization and connective tissue formation.

patient often presents a blind and painful eye, which may call for excision on account of the pain. At times, the fellow eye may also present glaucoma.

OPHTHALMOSCOPICALLY, incipient central venous occlusion is recognized by engorgement and tortuosity of the retinal veins, sometimes associated with a slight localized retinal edema, small retinal hemorrhages and some swelling of the optic disc. This ophthalmoscopic picture may precede the onset of central venous occlusion for a period varying from weeks to even months. The fully developed picture of occlusion of the central retinal vein (Figs. 222—225) is characterized by extensive flame-shaped, superficial retinal hemorrhages, and small, rounded, deep retinal hemorrhages, engorgement of the veins, swollen optic disc, fluffy exudates and edema throughout the fundus. The hemorrhages are larger near the disc than elsewhere. At times they break into the vitreous or form a preretinal hemorrhage. The veins are dark-red, dilated and tortuous. The arteries are usually narrow. The disc is red and swollen and the margin is blurred. Fluffy exudates may be present anywhere, but most frequently around the disc.

Recanalization of the vein is likely to occur in the course of some months, and hemorrhages and exudates tend to be absorbed. During that period, the retinal vessels usually become narrowed (Fig. 226), appear sclerotic and may sometimes be accompanied by pale sheaths, or be completely sheathed over a shorter or longer distance. Diffuse or patchy retinal atrophy is usually present. New-formed vascular channels sometimes develop a collateral circulation at or around the optic disc (Figs. 227, 236). In the late stage, bands or veils of connective tissue may also appear, preferentially around the disc area (Fig. 227). If glaucoma develops, glaucomatous atrophy of the disc may appear gradually.

The acute stage of central venous occlusion should not be confused with papilledema or hypertensive neuroretinopathy.

In branch vein occlusion, which is much more common than central vein occlusion, the visual symptoms depend on the site of the obstruction. If the macular area is involved, central vision is decreased or even lost. If a nasal branch is affected, however, there may be no symptoms at all. Secondary glaucoma is a rare complication in branch vein occlusion.

OPHTHALMOSCOPICALLY, an incipient branch vein occlusion is recognized by engorgement and tortuosity of a retinal vein (Fig. 230). In established occlusion of a branch of the central retinal vein (Figs. 231—233), the fundus changes, consisting of large superficial retinal hemorrhages and some cotton-wool exudates, are confined to a fan-shaped area drained by the obstructed vein. The occlusion is likely to develop at an arterio-

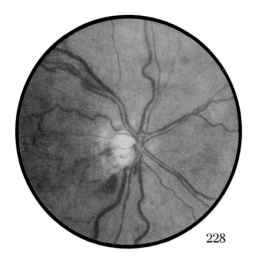

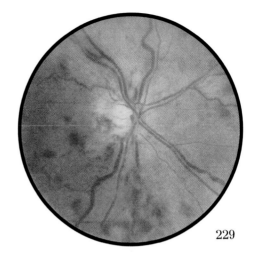

228

*Right eye. Commencing multiple retinal branch vein occlusions.*

229

*Same eye as figure 228, a week later, presents multiple branch vein occlusions.*

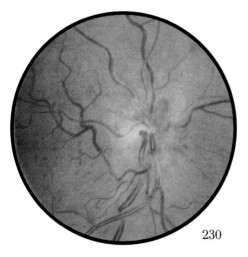

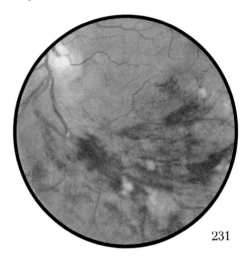

230

*Right eye. Commencing retinal branch vein occlusion.*

231

*Left eye. Retinal branch vein occlusion, acute stage.*

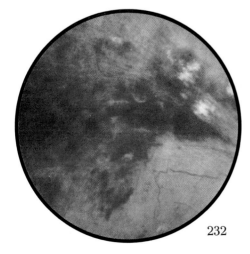

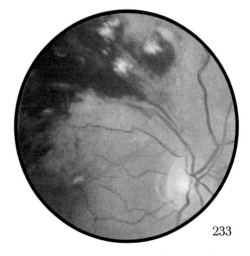

232

233

*Figures 232 and 233. Same right eye. Retinal branch vein occlusion. Peripheral to the occlusion*

*there are flame-shaped retinal hemorrhages and cotton-wool exudates.*

venous crossing, and most commonly affects the upper temporal vein. Multiple branch vein occlusions may also occur (Figs. 228—229).

The retinal hemorrhages and the exudates tend to be absorbed in the course of some months, although numerous small round red dots, probably clusters of microaneurysms, may remain in the diseased area for a long period (Fig. 234). Ensheathing of retinal veins is often present in late stages of venous occlusion (Figs. 237—239). New-formed vascular channels sometimes develop a collateral circulation (Fig. 235). This collateral circulation starts as a fine network of dilated capillary vessels, gradually acquiring the form of a unipolar rete mirabile, which is subsequently transformed into a bipolar rete mirabile. Finally, it assumes the simple form of an anastomosis, consisting of a single large vascular communication.

The late stage of branch vein occlusion should not be confused with diabetic retinopathy.

In central retinal vein occlusion and branch vein occlusion, alterations in the retinal blood circulation can readily be followed by fluorescein angiography.

Histopathologically, the central retinal vein may be obstructed by a thrombus or occluded by endothelial or subendothelial proliferations at or just behind the lamina cribrosa, and the condition is often accompanied by an atheromatous process in the central retinal artery. When coming to histopathological examination, however, the central retinal vein has often become recanalized, and the condition may then be indicated only by a finely perforated septum in the lumen of the vein, which is detectable in serial sections only.

In the early stages, the retinal changes are dominated by hemorrhages and edema. In the late stages, there is pronounced atrophy and disorganization of the retinal layers, marked gliosis, and sometimes preretinal, new-formed vessels and connective tissue.

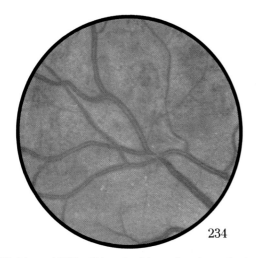

234

*Right eye (15°). Old retinal branch vein occlusion with microaneurysms.*

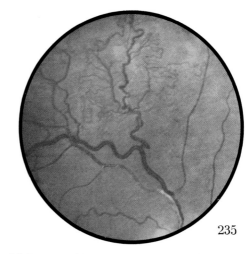

235

*Right eye. Old retinal branch vein occlusion with new vessel formation.*

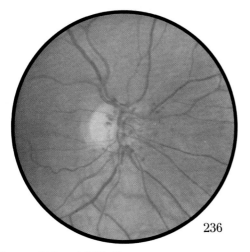

236

*Figures 236 and 237. Same right eye. Old retinal branch vein occlusion. At the disc, there is a small*

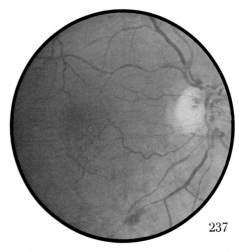

237

*tuft of new-formed vessels. A rete mirabile is seen below the fovea.*

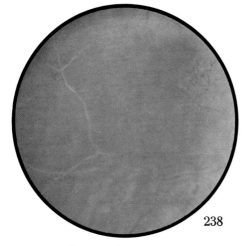

238

*Same eye as figures 236 and 237. In the perimacular area, the vessels are totally ensheathed.*

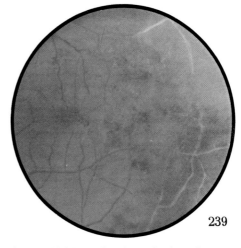

239

*Left eye. Old branch vein occlusion. Some retinal vessels ensheathed in the perimacular area.*

# Fundus and Vitreous Hemorrhage

(Figures 186—188, 222—224, 240—245, 247, 255, 259, 278—279, 282—283, 287—291, 352—353, 366 and 368—370)

Fundus hemorrhage may appear as superficial or deep retinal hemorrhage, subretinal hemorrhage, preretinal hemorrhage or, if a hemorrhage bursts through the hyaloid membrane, as vitreous hemorrhage.

Fundus hemorrhage may occur in various conditions such as retinal vascular obstruction, retinal perivasculitis, papilledema, subarachnoidal hemorrhage, vascular disease such as arteriosclerosis, different retinopathies, particularly diabetic and hypertensive, diseases of the hematopoetic system or following trauma. Finally, fundus hemorrhage is not infrequent in the new-born due to trauma of the head and neck during normal labor or due to instrumental delivery.

Whether visual disturbances occur or not, and whether they are major or minor, depend on the size and the localization of the fundus hemorrhage. In vitreous hemorrhage, however, vision is always decreased to some extent.

OPHTHALMOSCOPICALLY, retinal hemorrhages vary according to the localization of the blood. If the retinal hemorrhage is superficial, lying in the nerve-fiber layer, it assumes a striated or flame-shaped appearance (Figs. 186—188, 222—224, 278—279, 282—283), while hemorrhages in the deeper part of the retina are rounded or irregularly shaped, and usually smaller than superficial hemorrhages (Figs. 247, 287—291).

Subretinal hemorrhages appear most frequently around the optic disc or in the macular area.

OPHTHALMOSCOPICALLY, they are seen as ill-defined, dark-red, slate-gray or even black hemorrhages of disc size or even larger, lying beneath the retinal vessels (Figs. 244—245, 352—353, 366, 368—370).

Ophthalmoscopically, the condition may sometimes be difficult to separate from a commencing malignant choroidal melanoma. The lesions, however, can be distinguished by fluorescein angiography as a subretinal hemorrhage shows no fluorescence, while a malignant choroidal melanoma shows a characteristic pattern of fluorescence.

OPHTHALMOSCOPICALLY, a preretinal hemorrhage is seen as a dark-red or nearly black mass in front of the retina (Figs. 240—243, 255). The upper border is usually horizontal or slightly concave, while the lower is as a rule convex.

At times, both retinal, preretinal and subretinal hemorrhages may all be present simultaneously, either originating in the retina or subretinally, and then penetrating into the other layers (Figs. 244—245).

Any retinal or preretinal hemorrhage which is sufficiently profuse may burst into the vitreous, producing diffuse haze of the vitreous, forming clots floating

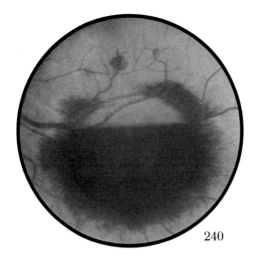

240

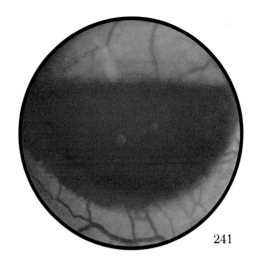

241

*Left eye. Large preretinal hemorrhage.*

*Right eye. Large preretinal hemorrhage in the macular area.*

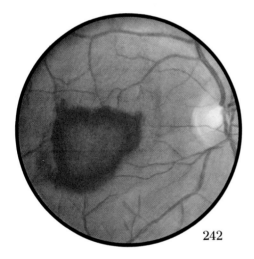

242

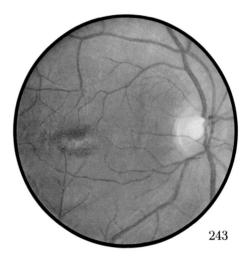

243

*Same eye as figure 241, nine weeks later. The hemorrhage is in absorption.*

*Same eye as figure 242, five weeks later. The hemorrhage has disappeared.*

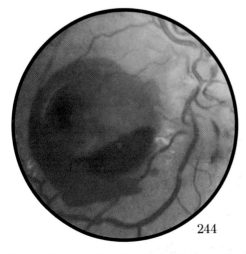

244

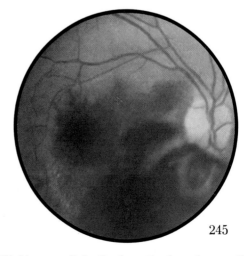

245

*Right eye. Preretinal and subretinal hemorrhage in the macular area.*

*Right eye. Subretinal, retinal and preretinal hemorrhages.*

around in the vitreous (Fig. 259) or being so large that it fills the whole vitreous with blood, giving rise to a dark-red or nearly black reflex in the pupil.

In the differential diagnosis of vitreous hemorrhage, it is necessary to consider for example angiomatosis of the retina, Eales' disease, diabetic retinopathy, malignant choroidal melanoma and retinal detachment.

Fundal and vitreous hemorrhages may be absorbed very quickly, but sometimes they may persist for months or even years, giving rise to fundal degeneration or development of proliferative retino-pathy.

HISTOPATHOLOGICALLY, superficial retinal hemorrhages lie in the nerve fiber layer while deep retinal hemorrhages lie in the outer and inner nuclear layers. Some degenerative changes are always present together with some glial proliferation. Subretinal hemorrhages lie between the choroid and the retinal pigment epithelium, often penetrating Bruch's membrane. Preretinal hemorrhages often lie behind the internal limiting membrane, which is detached from the nerve fiber layer, or penetrate the internal limiting membrane but remain behind the vitreous corpus.

# Diabetic Retinopathy
### (Figures 246—275)

Diabetes mellitus is probably that disease in which the most variegated picture of ocular complications or signs may be seen. These include retinopathy, cataract, changes in refraction, optic neuritis, lipemia retinalis, eye muscle palsies, rubeosis iridis and secondary glaucoma.

Diabetic retinopathy—which may be grouped into two main types, the simple and the proliferative retinopathy—is the ocular lesion which occurs most frequently. Like nephropathy, neuropathy, and cardiovascular changes, retinopathy is a late complication in diabetes and part of the diabetic angiopathy.

For many years, the incidence of diabetic retinopathy has been steadily increasing in all age-groups, particularly due to the increased longevity of diabetics since the introduction of insulin therapy.

In juveniles, diabetic retinopathy is never present when diabetes is demonstrated, and it occurs rarely before the age of 16 to 18 years, no matter how long the disease has lasted. In the older diabetics, however, retinopathy may be observed even before diabetes has been recognized clinically, although the diabetic state must have been present for years.

The incidence of retinopathy rises slowly during the first five years of diabetes, and more slowly in the younger age-groups than in the older age-groups. Then follows a sudden rise in incidence, and after about 10 years' duration, the

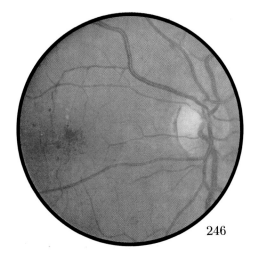

246

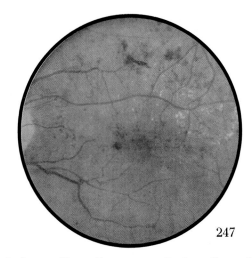

247

*Right eye. Simple diabetic retinopathy in a young diabetic, early stage.*

*Left eye. From the same patient as figure 246. Retinopathy more advanced.*

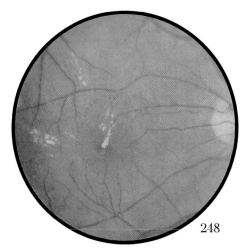

248

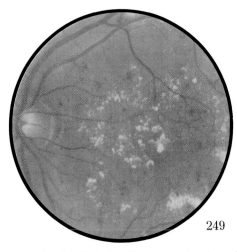

249

*Right eye in young diabetic. Some hard exudates and few microaneurysms.*

*Left eye in old diabetic. Numerous hard exudates and some microaneurysms.*

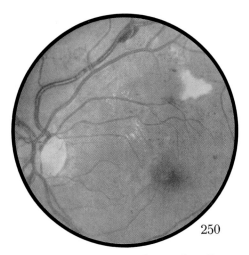

250

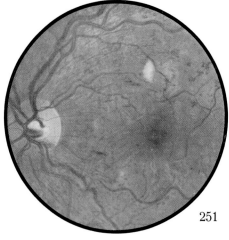

251

*Left eye. Simple retinopathy and cotton-wool exudates in a young diabetic.*

*Left eye. Rubeosis of the retina in diabetic retinopathy.*

incidence is nearly equal in all age-groups. After at least 15 years' duration, the incidence ranges from about 30 to 80 per cent, being lower in well controlled than in poorly controlled diabetics.

The incidence of diabetic retinopathy of the proliferative type has also shown a steady increase. In large series the incidence ranges from 2 to 8 per cent. Proliferative retinopathy is more frequent in the juvenile and middle-age groups than in the older age-groups. The average duration of diabetes before proliferative retinopathy develops, is 17 to 18 years in the younger age-groups and somewhat less in the older age-groups.

Various attempts have been made to classify diabetic retinopathy into different stages. It seems, however, more reasonable to consider diabetic retinopathy as two main types of retinopathy, the simple and the proliferative types, with a pre-proliferative stage interposed, and to consider the proliferative type not only as a progression of the simple type, but as a condition superimposed on the simple type.

Of the two main types of diabetic retinopathy, the simple type presents fundus changes such as venous dilatation, retinal microaneurysms, retinal hemorrhages and exudates, sclerosis of the retinal vessels and sometimes sheathing of the vessels. The proliferative type presents formation of new-formed vessels and fibrous tissue in the fundus. The pre-proliferative stage, which is a warning of transition from the simple to the proliferative type of diabetic retinopathy, is characterized by marked venous changes, preretinal hemorrhages, degenerative changes in the hyaloid membrane, vitreous detachment and vitreous hemorrhage.

Although the retinopathy is still progressive, there is nevertheless a tendency for periodic remissions and exacerbations.

Visual disturbances may be present or not, depending on the size and the localization of the fundus lesions. If the retinal lesions are not localized in or around the macula, vision may remain unaltered for many years, but in cases dominated by confluent exudates in the macular area, which occurs most often in mature onset diabetes, vision is often reduced at an early stage. Generally, however, the visual prognosis in simple diabetic retinopathy is fairly good.

When retinopathy proceeds to the pre-proliferative or proliferative stage, reduction or loss of vision will follow.

In the proliferative type of diabetic retinopathy, emphasis should be paid to the site of the neovascularization, because new-formed vessels extending from the disc have a poorer prognosis than new-formed vessels occurring in the fundus periphery. Furthermore, attention should be drawn to vitreous detachment associated with neovascularization on the posterior surface of the hyaloid membrane, as such cases usually have a poor visual prognosis.

In the individual case of simple diabetic retinopathy it may be difficult or impossible ophthalmoscopically to evaluate if the retinopathy will continue as the simple type of diabetic retinopathy or

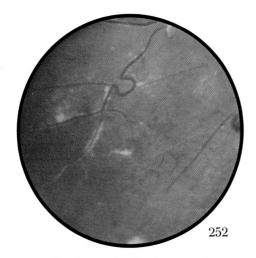

252

*Left eye. Sheathing of retinal vessels in diabetic retinopathy.*

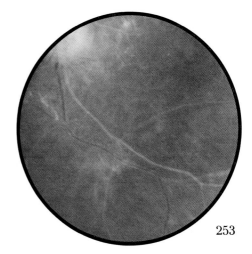

253

*Left eye. Heavy sheathing of retinal vessels in diabetic retinopathy.*

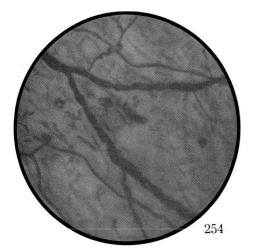

254

*Right eye (15°). Advanced phlebopathy in diabetic retinopathy.*

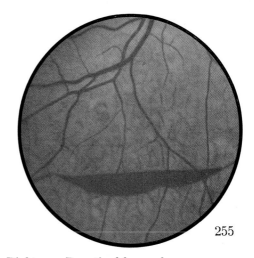

255

*Right eye. Preretinal hemorrhage.*

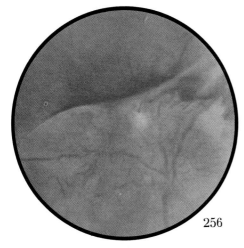

256

*Left eye. Vitreous detachment. Retrovitreal space filled with hemorrhagic fluid.*

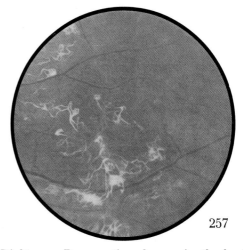

257

*Right eye. Degenerative changes in the hyaloid membrane.*

later on will show a transition from the simple to the proliferative type of diabetic retinopathy.

In these cases, a determination of the oscillatory potential in the b-wave of the electroretinogram may be of prognostic value. If the oscillatory potential is diminished or abolished, this is a warning of transition from the simple to the proliferative type of diabetic retinopathy.

Even if the number of diabetics with diabetic retinopathy is very large and the number of diabetics showing visual disturbances is very small, **diabetic retinopathy is now the major or one of the most important causes of acquired blindness in many countries.**

OPHTHALMOSCOPICALLY, the earliest fundus changes in simple diabetic retinopathy (Figs. 246—249) are mostly situated in the posterior part of the fundus. They consist of scattered microaneurysms, punctate retinal hemorrhages and some venous dilatation. In older diabetics, sharply outlined exudates are also often present in the early stage of retinopathy. In juvenile diabetics, however, they are seldom present at this stage.

Retinal microaneurysms (Figs. 246, 247, 249) are seen ophthalmoscopically as small, round, distinctly outlined, dark-red or nearly black spots, often with a central reflex. Their diameter is usually less than one half of the diameter of a large vein. Punctate retinal hemorrhages are seen as rounded red spots, often closely resembling microaneurysms.

In a single ophthalmoscopic examination, it is often difficult to distinguish microaneurysms from deep punctate hemorrhages, but repeated examinations show that microaneurysms remain unchanged for long periods, whereas hemorrhages tend to be absorbed quickly. However, the distinction is easily made by fluorescein angiography, since the aneurysms fluoresce while the hemorrhages do not fluoresce. As new retinal hemorrhages develop and disappear simultaneously, the general ophthalmoscopic picture is often maintained.

Diabetic exudates (Figs. 248—249) consist of minute white or yellowish-white, well-defined flecks, of the same size as microaneurysms or punctate retinal hemorrhages, tending to coalesce into larger irregular patches. In long-standing diabetes, woolly exudates may occur in association with or without hypertension or nephropathy (Figs. 250—251).

As the diabetic retinopathy proceeds, the number of microaneurysms increases, the retinal hemorrhages enlarge in size and number, and superficial retinal hemorrhages sometimes develop. The exudates tend to be more numerous and to coalesce into larger, irregular, white or yellowish-white patches, or into large, glistening, waxy-looking masses, or tend to be arranged in a circinate manner.

In advanced retinopathy, the retinal vessels may show a varying degree of sclerosis and sheathing of the retinal vessels (Figs. 252—253), and the fundus picture is often altered by the presence of hypertensive fundus changes.

The development of proliferative retinopathy is preceded or followed by marked

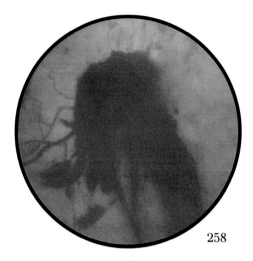

258

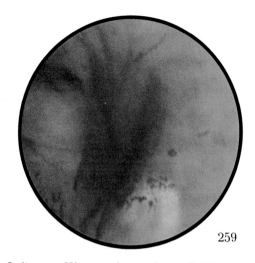

259

*Right eye. Preretinal hemorrhage with extension into the vitreous.*

*Left eye. Vitreous hemorrhage. Outlines of the disc are seen faintly.*

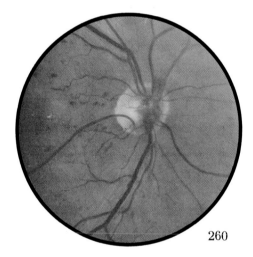

260

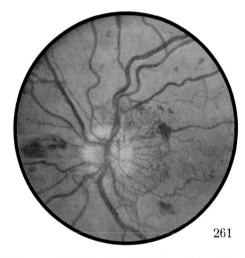

261

*Right eye. Proliferative diabetic retinopathy. Prepapillary tuft of new-formed vessels.*

*Left eye. Proliferative diabetic retinopathy with prepapillary neovascularization.*

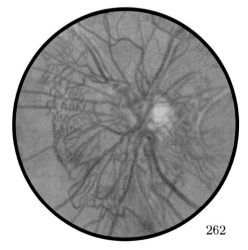

262

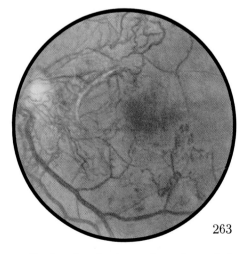

263

*Figures 262 and 263. Same left eye. Proliferative diabetic retinopathy with extensive fan-shaped*

*preretinal network of new-formed vessels leaving the macular area free.*

variations in caliber of the retinal veins, often giving the veins an appearance of a string of sausages (Fig. 254), by pre-retinal hemorrhages (Figs. 255, 258), degenerative changes in the hyaloid membrane (Fig. 257), vitreous detachment (Fig. 256) and vitreous hemorrhage (Fig. 259).

Proliferative diabetic retinopathy is characterized by the formation of new-formed vessels and fibrous tissue in the fundus or by one of these changes only.

The new-formed vessels and fibrous tissue may develop anywhere in the fundus.

Ophthalmoscopically, the new-formed vessels extending from the disc (Figs. 260—266) are seen as small tufts of vessels lying in a delicate stroma and protruding forwards, waving to-and-fro when the eye is moved, or extending pre-retinally towards the periphery. When they occur in the fundal periphery (Figs. 267—268), the new-formed vessels lie pre-retinally in tufts or fan-shaped figures, closely apposed to the retina on the posterior side of the hyaloid membrane. In most instances they retain the position unaltered when the eye is moved, but in vitreous detachment they follow the detached membrane, so that when the eye is moved, they wave to-and-fro.

In the course of time the new-formed vessels may show some atrophy and the delicate supporting stroma of the neovascularization is converted into fibrous tissue. However, new vascular proliferations may often develop at the border of the lesion, and hemorrhages, especially vitreous hemorrhage, may accelerate this process.

Fibrous tissue (Figs. 269—272) is seen as preretinal white or grayish-white veils or membranes, fibrous bands or solid masses, covering smaller or larger areas of the fundus. Following vitreous hemorrhage, fibrous tissue may develop in the vitreous. When the fibrous tissue contracts in the course of time, the retina is detached (Figs. 273—275).

By means of fluorescein angiography it is possible to follow closely the vascular alterations throughout the various stages of diabetic retinopathy.

In the late stage of diabetic retinopathy, rubeosis iridis and hemorrhagic glaucoma may develop. In these cases, the patient often presents a blind and painful eye, calling for excision on account of the pain.

Histopathologically, the characteristic changes in simple diabetic retinopathy consist of microaneurysms, retinal hemorrhages and exudates. The microaneurysms are found on the venous side of the capillary network and mainly in the inner nuclear layer. They are sharply outlined, mulberry-like globules measuring 30 to 90 microns. Their walls are often thickened and contain deposits of hyaline PAS-positive material. The hemorrhages are mainly found in the outer plexiform and nuclear layers. The exudates lie in the same layers as the hemorrhages, and consist of albuminous, hyaline and fatty material. The retinal vessels show a varying degree of arteriolosclerosis, phlebosclerosis, and capillary sclerosis, resulting from deposits

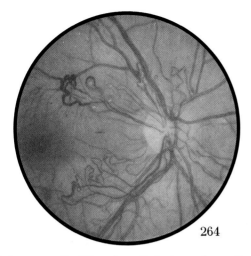

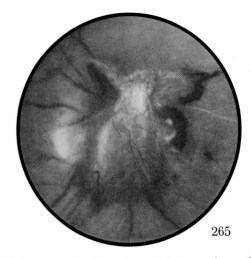

264

*Right eye. Proliferative diabetic retinopathy. Preretinal neovascularization.*

265

*Right eye. Proliferative diabetic retinopathy. Fibrous tissue and new-formed vessels.*

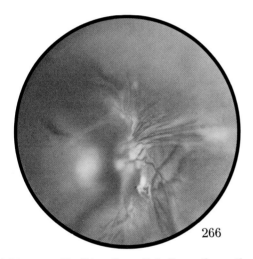

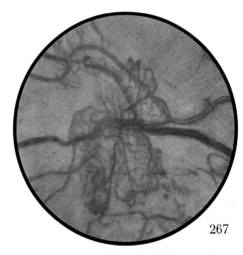

266

*Right eye. Proliferative diabetic retinopathy. Neovascularization and fibrous tissue.*

267

*Right eye (15°). Proliferative diabetic retinopathy. Preretinal neovascularization.*

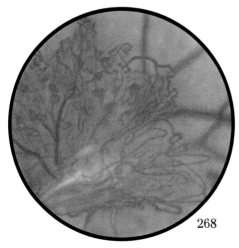

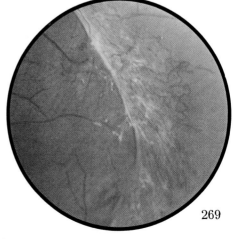

268

*Left eye (15°). Proliferative diabetic retinopathy. Preretinal neovascularization.*

269

*Right eye. Proliferative diabetic retinopathy. Preretinal fibrous tissue veil.*

of PAS-positive hyaline material in the vessel walls.

The histological picture in proliferative diabetic retinopathy is very complex, showing intraretinal new-formed channels and preretinal or prepapillary networks of new-formed vessels, sometimes piercing the internal limiting membrane and occupying a smaller or larger part of the vitreous. The new-formed vessels are supported in a delicate matrix of connective tissue, often transformed here and there into solid fibrous strands or masses, resulting in retinal detachment.

# Lipemia Retinalis
### (Figures 276—277)

Lipemia retinalis is a rare condition due to a marked elevation of the serum lipids, either triglycerides or cholesterol or both. It occurs most often in xanthomatosis and in diabetic acidosis.

OPHTHALMOSCOPICALLY, the fundus (Figs. 276—277) appears slightly indistinct and lighter red than normal, due to a vitreous haze and accumulation of lipids in the retinal tissue. The color of the retinal vessels varies from salmon-pink to almost milky-white, and the vessels sometimes assume a ribbon-like appearance. The vascular light reflex is less brilliant than normal or may even disappear, and sometimes it may be difficult or impossible to distinguish the retinal vessels from the fundus background.

HISTOPATHOLOGICALLY, there is an accumulation of lipid in the retinal vessels and the perivascular tissue.

# Fundus Changes in Anemia
### (Figures 278—279)

Fundus changes may occur in all types of anemia, including macrocytic, microcytic and aplastic anemia, when the hemoglobin level falls to 6.0 g/100 ml or below. Evident fundus changes are therefore uncommon in anemia, and are most frequently observed in untreated cases of pernicious anemia.

Vision is not altered unless the macula is involved or optic atrophy develops.

OPHTHALMOSCOPICALLY, the fundus changes (Figs. 278—279) consist of superficial flame-shaped hemorrhages, often with a small fluffy whitish center, small rounded deep retinal hemorrhages, and some cotton-wool exudates. These lesions are mainly located around the disc. The retinal arteries are pale and the veins often dilated. The fundus may show a varying degree of pallor and not infre-

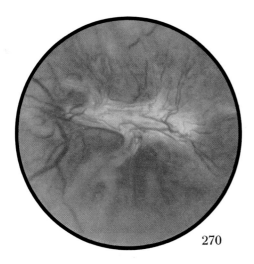

270

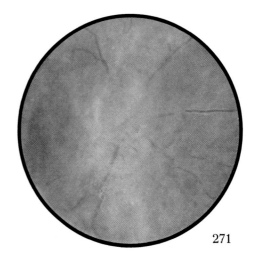

271

*Right eye. Proliferative diabetic retinopathy. Preretinal mass of fibrous tissue.*

*Right eye. Proliferative diabetic retinopathy. Preretinal veil of fibrous tissue.*

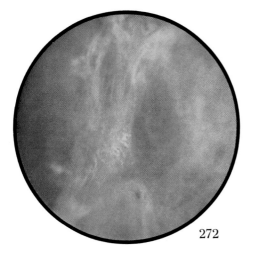

272

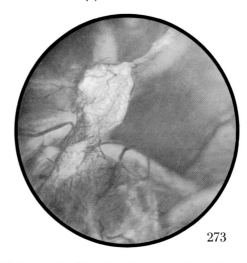

273

*Right eye. Proliferative diabetic retinopathy. Preretinal veil of fibrous tissue.*

*Right eye. Proliferative diabetic retinopathy with retinal detachment.*

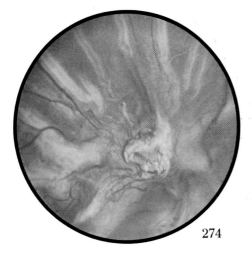

274

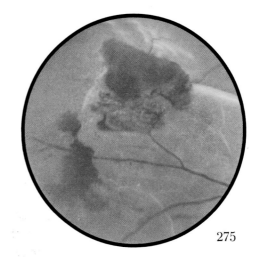

275

*Same eye as figure 273. Proliferative tissue on top of detached retina.*

*Same eye as figures 273 and 274. Retinal tear partly covered by hemorrhage.*

quently slight edema. The optic disc may be normal or show some pallor. In advanced cases papilledema may be present, and eventually optic atrophy may develop.

It is not possible from the ophthalmoscopic picture to differentiate the various forms of anemia.

## Polycythemia
### (Figures 280—281)

Polycythemia is a condition characterized by a marked increase of red blood cells. The condition may be primary, as in polycythemia vera, or secondary as in congenital heart disease, severe pulmonary insufficiency or pulmonary vascular sclerosis. Both types, however, cause similar fundus changes.

Visual disturbances may occur as muscae volitantes and scotomas, and profound visual disturbances occur if the condition is complicated by retinal venous occlusion.

OPHTHALMOSCOPICALLY, the fundus in polycythemia (Figs. 280—281) has a deep-red color. The retinal vessels and especially the veins appear engorged and tortuous and the color is darker red than normal. The disc is hyperemic and may show a varying degree of edema. Retinal hemorrhages and exudates are usually absent or few in number, unless retinal venous thrombosis is present.

HISTOPATHOLOGICALLY, the retinal vessels are dilated, retinal hemorrhages may be present, and the optic disc may show a varying degree of edema.

## Leukemia
### (Figures 97 and 282—283)

All types of leukemia may present fundus lesions. The lesions are indistinguishable from one another and may occur at any stage of the disease, but are seen most frequently in acute leukemia, in late stages of chronic leukemia and in periods of severe anemia.

Visual disturbances occur only when the macula is involved, or when vitreous hemorrhage is present.

OPHTHALMOSCOPICALLY, the fundus lesions (Figs. 282—283) consist of retinal hemorrhages of varying size and shape, and frequently contain a fluffy whitish patch centrally. Whitish woolly exudates or infiltrates of varying size may be present in the posterior part of the fundus. Retinal microaneurysms may also occur. The retinal veins are frequently tortuous and dilated, and sometimes appear like a string of sausages or show pronounced sheathing. The fundus color often remains normal until the late stages, when fundus and retinal vessels become more orange-colored. At times the disc margin is slightly blurred and occasionally more pronounced papilledema is present, especially in children with intracranial leukemic infiltrations (Fig. 97).

The retinal hemorrhages with a pale

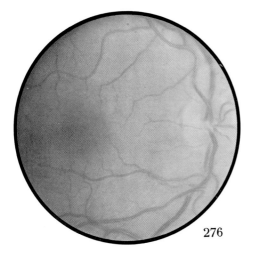

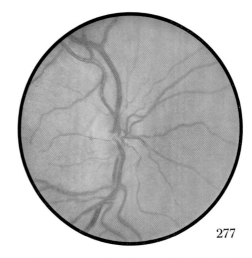

276

277

*Figures 276 and 277. Same right eye. Lipemia retinalis. The fundus is pale and the retinal*   vessels have a nearly salmon-pink color. Blurring caused by vitreous haze.

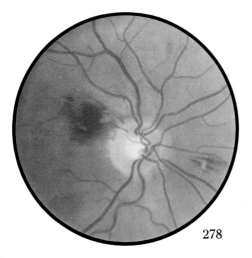

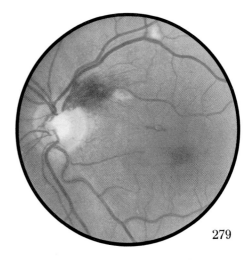

278

279

*Figures 278 and 279. Right and left eyes. Retinopathy in anemia. Flame-shaped retinal*   hemorrhages and some cotton-wool exudates are seen in both fundi.

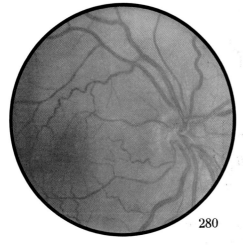

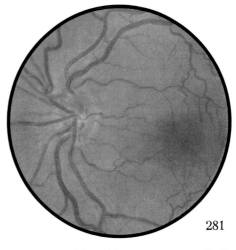

280

281

*Figures 280 and 281. Right and left eyes. Fundus changes in polycythemia. The retinal vessels,*   optic discs and fundi have assumed a darker red color than normal.

center are characteristic of leukemia but not pathognomonic, and may also occur in conditions such as severe anemias, including pernicious anemia, and septicemias, including subacute bacterial endocarditis.

Histopathologically, white blood cells may infiltrate the retina and accumulate in the perivascular areas. Hemorrhages and exudates may be present throughout the retina.

# Myelomatosis or Multiple Myeloma
(Figures 99 and 284—287)

Myelomatosis or multiple myeloma is a rare, malignant disease of the reticuloendothelial system characterized by widespread infiltration of the bone marrow throughout the body. The principal cell type in these infiltrates is the plasma cell.

Neurological symptoms, pain and a very high sedimentation rate are usually present. Hyperproteinemia occurs in many cases, with reversal of the normal albumin-globulin ratio, and paraproteins are often present as well as secondary anemia. In about 50 per cent of the cases, Bence-Jones protein is found in the urine. The skeletal lesions are seen radiologically mainly as round, well-defined bone defects.

Fundus lesions are uncommon. Unless the macula is involved, there are no visual disturbances.

Ophthalmoscopically, the most common lesions (Fig. 284) are superficial retinal hemorrhages and cotton-wool exudates located mainly around the optic disc.

In cases associated with paraproteinemia, the fundus changes may be much more pronounced (Figs. 285—287), showing a similarity with those changes found in macroglobulinemia. The veins are engorged and tortuous, and sometimes appear like a string of sausages. Small and large, rounded or streaky retinal hemorrhages are seen all over the fundus. In some areas the fundus is pale and yellowish due to retinal or subretinal exudation. Papilledema (Fig. 99) may also be present.

# Macroglobulinemia (Waldenström)
(Figures 98 and 288—291)

Macroglobulinemia, which belongs to the dys- or paraproteinemias, is a rare, chronic condition characterized by purpura or bleeding from the mucous membranes of the nose and gums, some enlargement of the lymph nodes, and often enlargement of the liver and spleen. Neurological symptoms may sometimes be present.

There is a normochromic anemia and a markedly increased sedimentation rate. The serum is viscous, the total protein content high, the serum albumin lowered and the serum globulins dominated by a component of high-molecular weight, known as macroglobulin or the 20-S component. The platelet adhesivity is zero *in vivo,* but it is normal *in vitro.*

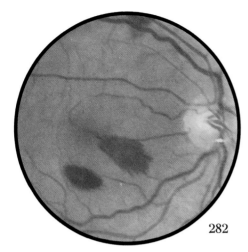

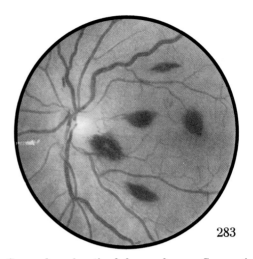

*Figures 282 and 283. Right and left eyes. Fundus changes in leukemia, consisting of* *flame-shaped retinal hemorrhages. Some of the hemorrhages have a fluffy whitish center.*

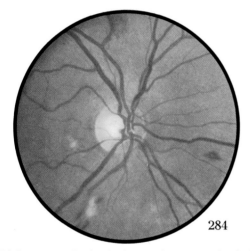

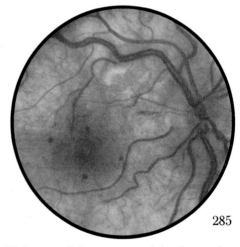

*Right eye. Retinal hemorrhages and fluffy exudates in myelomatosis.*

*Right eye. Pale, orange-red fundus and swollen disc in myelomatosis.*

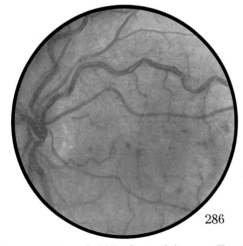

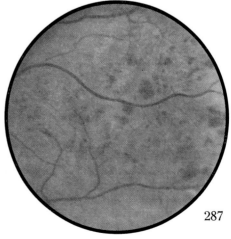

*Figures 286 and 287. Same left eye. Fundus changes in myelomatosis. Retinal veins are* *engorged. Numerous hemorrhages and micro-aneurysms in fundus periphery.*

Characteristic fundus changes may occur in the course of the disease, and especially in cases with neurological symptoms.

Visual disturbances may be present or not, depending on the site and extension of the fundus lesions. When the lesions are extensive, secondary glaucoma may develop.

OPHTHALMOSCOPICALLY, the fundus lesions are characterized by venous changes, retinal hemorrhages, microaneurysms (Figs. 288—291), retinal or subretinal exudation, and sometimes by papilledema (Fig. 98).

The retinal veins are engorged and tortuous. Localized venous constrictions are often present, in some places giving the veins an appearance resembling a string of beads or sausages. Small or large, rounded and streaky retinal hemorrhages are seen all over the fundus but often most numerous in the fundus periphery.

Clusters of small red dots, probably accumulations of microaneurysms, are often seen as red patches together with the hemorrhages. In some areas the fundus may be pale and yellowish due to retinal or subretinal exudation (Fig. 98). Fluffy exudates, however, are not characteristic. Papilledema often occurs in cases with involvement of the central nervous system.

Similar fundus changes may occur in cryoglobulinemia and other paraproteinemias.

The condition should not be confused with occlusion of the central retinal vein or diabetic retinopathy.

HISTOPATHOLOGICALLY, the veins are dilated and the retina presents hemorrhages and microaneurysms. Retinal and subretinal exudates may also be present, and the optic disc may show varying degrees of edema.

## Collagen Diseases
(Figures 292—293)

The collagen diseases are a group of diseases characterized by widespread alteration of the ground substance resulting in fibrinoid necrosis. These diseases are probably related to hypersensitivity or autoimmunity.

Cutaneous eruptions, joint pain, low-grade fever and hypertension are some of the characteristic clinical symptoms.

Among the collagen diseases, fundus changes are most often observed in polyarteritis nodosa, disseminated lupus erythematosus, dermatomyositis, scleroderma and anaphylactoid purpura, while fundus changes have not been observed in conditions such as rheumatic fever and rheumatoid arthritis.

Visual disturbances do not occur unless the macula is involved.

OPHTHALMOSCOPICALLY, the fundus changes are characterized (Figs. 292—293) by more or less numerous fluffy exudates of varying size and sometimes superficial retinal hemorrhages, both located around the disc and in the posterior pole. Hypertensive fundus changes and vascular occlusions may alter the ophthalmoscopic picture. Thus, the ophthalmoscopic appearance is not pathognomonic in any of these diseases.

HISTOPATHOLOGICALLY, the conditions are characterized by inflammatory changes in the vessel walls, cytoid bodies and superficial retinal hemorrhages.

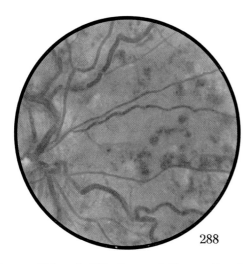

288

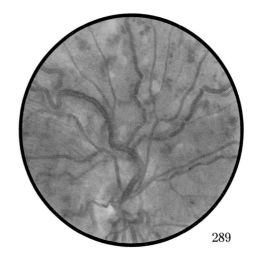

289

*Figures 288 and 289. Same right eye. Fundus changes in macroglobulinemia. Retinal veins are*

*engorged. Hemorrhages and microaneurysms are diffusely scattered in the fundus.*

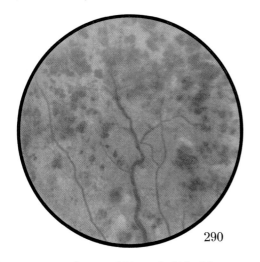

290

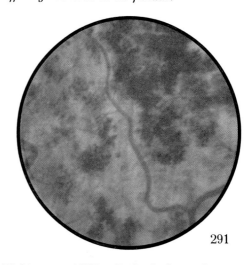

291

*Same eye as figures 288 and 289. Numerous hemorrhages and some microaneurysms.*

*Right eye (15°). Retinal hemorrhages and microaneurysms in macroglobulinemia.*

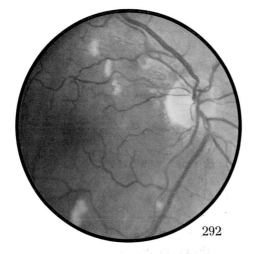

292

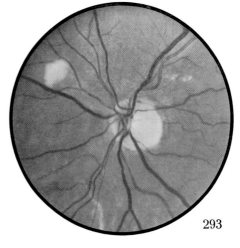

293

*Figures 292 and 293. Right and left eyes. Fundus changes in collagenosis. Both fundi present*

*several cotton-wool exudates. Retinal arteries are narrow, veins are normal.*

# Choroideremia
(Figures 294—295)

Choroideremia is a rare tapeto-choroidal dystrophy inherited in an intermediate sex-linked manner, presenting a progressive dystrophy in males and a non-progressive dystrophy in females.

In affected males the earliest and most prominent symptom is night blindness, which usually becomes evident during childhood and is later followed by a concentric contraction of the visual field. Central vision usually remains good until the age of about 40 years. After that time, central vision becomes gradually reduced. The electroretinographic response shows a gradual reduction and finally becomes extinguished.

Female carriers show no visual disturbances and visual fields and dark adaption remain normal.

OPHTHALMOSCOPICALLY, fundus changes in the affected males are seen in the earliest stage as a salt-and-pepper configuration. When this pigmentary atrophy progresses, the choroidal vessels become exposed in wide areas, but simultaneously the choroidal vessels show a progressive disappearance. When fully developed (Figs. 294—295), there is only a central patch of choroidal tissue left in the macular area while elsewhere the atrophic choroid is exposed, and small pigment deposits are scattered throughout the fundus. The optic disc remains normal, while the retinal vessels show some narrowing.

The condition should not be confused with primary choroidal atrophy.

In female carriers the ophthalmoscopic changes are limited to the peripheral salt-and-pepper configuration seen in the early stages of the affected males.

HISTOPATHOLOGICALLY, in the late stage the choroid, pigment epithelium and rods and cones are completely absent except in the macular area.

# Gyrate Atrophy of the Choroid and Retina
(Figures 296—297)

Gyrate atrophy is a rare, slowly progressive, heredodegenerative chorioretinal disease affecting both sexes equally.

The symptoms may commence during childhood or early adult life. The first symptom is usually the observation of night blindness, which is later followed by a progressive contraction of the visual field and a progressive reduction of vision. A progressive myopia is frequently present in these cases.

In early stages, the electroretinographic response is normal, later it becomes subnormal and finally extinguished.

OPHTHALMOSCOPICALLY, the condition usually commences in the fundal periphery with irregular or rounded, well-defined, more or less confluent areas of chorioretinal atrophy. As the condition progresses, wide areas of the fundus may be involved (Figs. 296—297), but the macula is usually spared. In the atrophic areas the exposed sclera has a whitish or yellowish-white color, the choroidal vessels are practically absent, and scattered clumps of retinal pigment are seen plain-

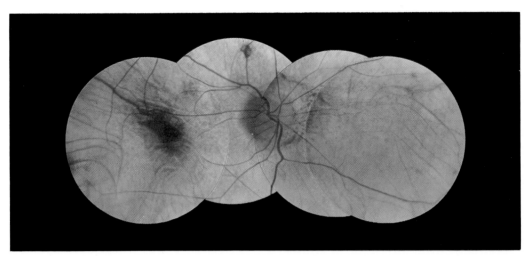

Figure 294. Composite picture. Right eye. Choroideremia. The fundus is pale, whitish with atrophy of the choroid and some choroidal pigment accumulation in the macula.

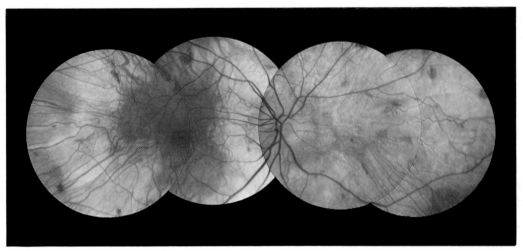

Figure 295. Composite picture. Right eye. Choroideremia. The choroid is intact in the macular area, but elsewhere it is atrophic. There are scattered clusters of pigment.

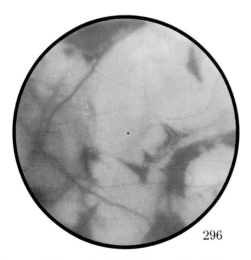

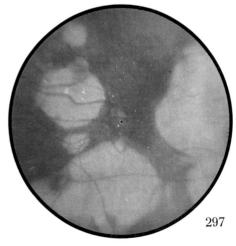

Figures 296 and 297. Left and right eyes. Gyrate atrophy of the choroid and retina. There are confluent chorioretinal atrophies and scattered pigment clumping.

ly. The retinal vessels appear normal or slightly contracted.

In the final stage the ophthalmoscopic appearance resembles to some extent that in choroideremia. Gyrate atrophy of the choroid must not be confused with primary choroidal atrophy.

# Retinitis Pigmentosa
### (Figures 298—301)

Retinitis pigmentosa or pigmentary retinal dystrophy is a degenerative disease of the retina, commencing in the retinal neuroepithelium, particularly in the rods.

The condition is characterized by widespread pigmentary changes in the retina, narrowing of the retinal vessels, optic atrophy, and is associated with night blindness and constriction of the visual fields. The electroretinographic response is markedly subnormal or completely extinguished at an early stage, while central vision becomes reduced in the late stage.

The disease is progressive and bilateral. A hereditary tendency is observed in about two-thirds of the cases, and in the majority of these the inheritance is recessive. The two sexes are affected almost equally. However, the condition may occur rarely in a sex-linked form. The incidence of retinitis pigmentosa is estimated at about five per 1,000 individuals.

The first symptom is night blindness, commonly noticed in childhood. As the disease progresses, a ring scotoma is produced, which increases gradually in a central and peripheral direction until it involves the whole peripheral field. Finally, the visual field shows a marked constriction, so that only tubular vision remains. When the visual field is reduced to about 10°, central vision also becomes markedly diminished.

The disease runs a variable course, but considerable disturbance of vision usually occurs in the thirties, leading to practical blindness in the forties and fifties. The condition is often associated with myopia, and cataract frequently develops in the course of the disease.

OPHTHALMOSCOPICALLY, there are no visible fundus changes in the early stages, but the electroretinographic response is markedly subnormal or completely extinguished. The earliest retinal changes are seen as scattered accumulations of dark-brown or black pigment, assuming a bone corpuscle configuration (Figs. 298—301). The initial pigment changes occur at the equator and progress towards the periphery and the macular area. The amount of pigment gradually increases, and in advanced cases pigment deposits are also arranged around the retinal vessels, the pigment sheathing of which becomes a characteristic feature of the disease. Depigmented areas are left in which the choroidal vessels are seen plainly. The retinal vessels show a marked narrowing (Fig. 301), and this may appear even before obvious pigmentary changes are present. The optic disc shows a progressive pallor and assumes a grayish or yellowish-gray color (Fig. 301). In the advanced stage, the macula may assume a moth-eaten appearance (Fig. 301).

In the typical case the diagnosis is not difficult. Atypical cases may occur, how-

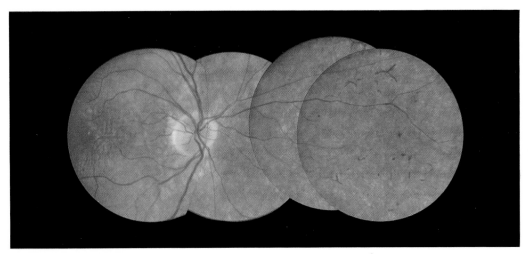

Figure 298. Composite picture, right eye. Retinitis pigmentosa. Typical bone corpuscle-like pigment deposits and some patchy atrophy in the fundus periphery.

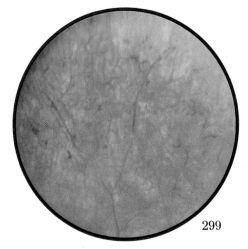

299

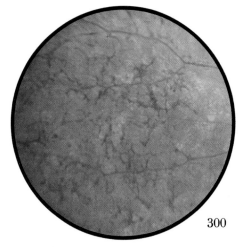

300

Same eye as figure 298. Pigment deposits and narrow retinal vessels.

Left eye. Retinitis pigmentosa. Bone corpuscle-like pigment deposits.

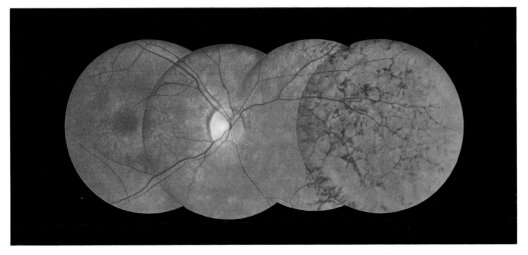

Figure 301. Composite picture. Right eye. From the same patient as figure 300. The optic dics is pale, retinal vessels narrow. Bone corpuscle-like pigment deposits nasally.

ever, with little or no pigment, abnormal pigment distribution or sectorial pigment accumulation. Even unilateral cases may occur. In all those cases the diagnosis is confirmed by the abnormal electroretinographic response. The condition must be distinguished from other degenerative fundus diseases, and also from disseminated choroiditis.

HISTOPATHOLOGICALLY, the condition is characterized by a disappearance of the retinal neuroepithelial cells, at first the rods and later the cones. Glial cells and pigment epithelium proliferate, and cellular strands of pigment epithelium migrate into the retinal tissue and frequently accumulate around the retinal vessels. The vessels show thickening of their walls and a diminished lumen. In the optic nerve the nerve fibers are often replaced by glial tissue, and a glial membrane is sometimes formed in front of the optic disc. The inner retinal layers rarely show severe changes until a late stage of the disease.

## Retinitis Punctata Albescens
### (Figures 302—305)

Retinitis punctata albescens or albipunctate dystrophy is a rare heredofamilial disease characterized by innumerable small white dots scattered over the fundus and associated with night blindness.

The condition occurs in a stationary and a progressive form.

The stationary form commences in childhood with night blindness, but vision, visual fields, color sense and usually also electroretinographic response remain normal.

OPHTHALMOSCOPICALLY, the fundus shows a multitude of minute white dots diffusely scattered in the fundus, leaving the macular area free. The disc and retinal vessels appear normal.

In the progressive form, night blindness is present from childhood. The visual fields show a progressive contraction and central vision gradually deteriorates. The electroretinographic response is subnormal or extinguished.

OPHTHALMOSCOPICALLY, the progressive form, like the stationary form, shows a multitude of minute white dots scattered in the fundus (Figs. 302—303, 305), but small pigment deposits (Fig. 303) often showing a bone corpuscle configuration may also be present. The retinal vessels show some narrowing and the optic disc some pallor (Fig. 304). At times the macular area is involved (Fig. 304), showing depigmentation and pigment accumulation.

## Fundus Flavimaculatus
### (Figures 306—307)

Fundus flavimaculatus is a rare, possibly congenital condition characterized by white or yellowish-white, irregular patches in the fundus, confined to the posterior pole and often associated with degenerative changes at the macula.

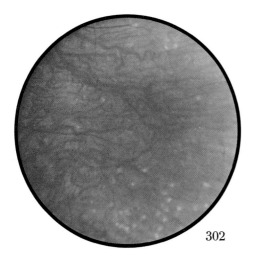

302

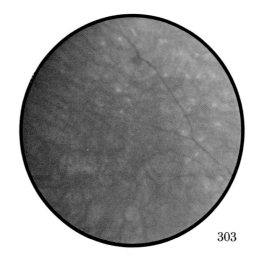

303

*Right eye. Albipunctate dystrophy with numerous small white dots.*

*Left eye. From the same patient as figure 302.*

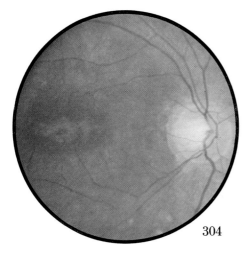

304

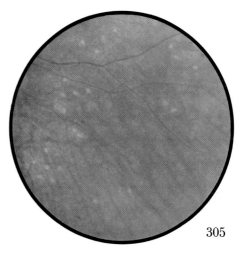

305

*Right eye. Macular changes and optic atrophy in albipunctate dystrophy.*

*From the same eye as figure 304. White dots in the fundus periphery.*

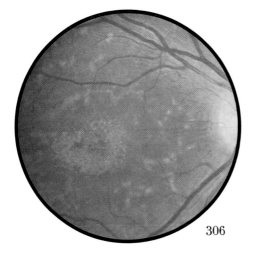

306

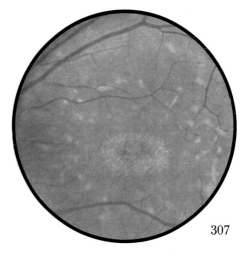

307

*Figures 306 and 307. Right and left eyes. Fundus flavimaculatus, seen as yellowish, irregular flecks*

*in the posterior pole. There is also some macular degeneration.*

Vision may be normal, but if the macula is involved central vision decreases. The visual fields are usually normal and the condition is seldom associated with night blindness. The electroretinographic response is usualy normal or subnormal.

Ophthalmoscopically, the condition is characterized (Figs. 306—307) by small or large, irregular, yellow or yellowish-white patches or lines mainly confined to the posterior pole. The macula may show degenerative changes, but the retinal vessels and the optic disc are normal.

In juvenile heredomacular degeneration (Figs. 324—325), fundus changes may occasionally occur similar to those seen in fundus flavimaculatus.

# Amaurotic Family Idiocy

(Figures 308—313)

Amaurotic family idiocy is a rare, recessive, familial disease belonging to the lipoidoses. It is characterized by degenerative changes in the retina and the central nervous system and accumulation of gangliosides in the ganglion cells in the central nervous system as well as in the retina.

It occurs in two types, the infantile, known as Tay-Sachs' disease and the juvenile, known as Spielmeyer-Vogt, Spielmeyer-Stock or Batten-Mayou's disease.

The infantile type, which is predominant among Jews, commences during the first year of life. It is rapidly progressive and death occurs usually within one or two years. It is characterized by the lack of mental development, progressive muscular weakness, paralyses, convulsions and rapidly developing blindness. The electroretinogram, however, is normal.

Ophthalmoscopically, both foveae are surrounded in the early stage by an opaque, whitish zone, not unlike that seen in central retinal artery occlusion, and the foveae are seen as cherry-red spots (Fig. 308). The disc and the retinal vessels appear normal. Later, however, the opacification clears somewhat, the cherry-red spots become less distinct, the discs atrophic and the retinal vessels narrow.

The condition should not be confused with occlusion of the central retinal artery, and it is distinguished from Niemann-Pick's disease and Gaucher's disease by the general clinical symptoms.

Histopathologically, there is diffuse lipoidal degeneration of the cytoplasm of the ganglion cells of the retina and the central nervous system, and the ganglion cells are PAS-positive and contain gangliosides.

In Niemann-Pick's disease, which is a rare congenital condition belonging to the lipoidoses and characterized by widespread deposits of sphingomyelin and possibly cerebrosides in the retina, the central nervous system and the viscera, particularly the liver and spleen, fundus changes may occur (Fig. 309) similar to those described in Tay-Sachs' disease, although not as frequently as in the latter disease.

A similar ophthalmoscopic picture has

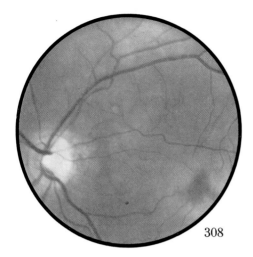

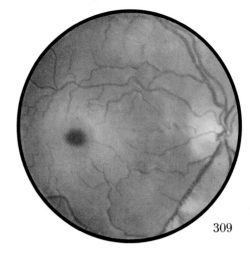

*Left eye. Tay-Sachs' disease. Disc is atrophic, fovea is deep red.*

*Right eye. Niemann-Pick's disease. The fovea presents a "cherry-red" spot.*

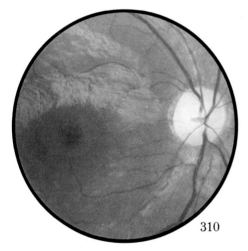

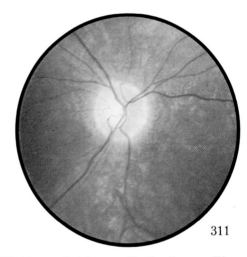

*Right eye. Spielmeyer-Vogt's disease, early stage. Disc pale. Pigment clumping in the fovea.*

*Right eye. Spielmeyer-Vogt's disease. The optic disc is atrophic.*

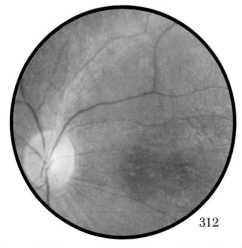

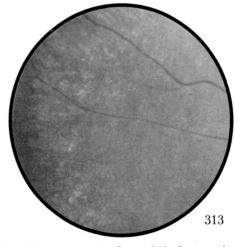

*Left eye. Spielmeyer-Vogt's disease. Disc is pale, retinal arteries narrow.*

*From the same eye as figure 312. Coarse pigmentation and depigmentation.*

been described in Gaucher's disease, which also belongs to the lipoidoses and is characterized by the accumulation of cerebrosides, mainly in the reticulo-endothelial system.

THE JUVENILE TYPE of amaurotic family idiocy, also belonging to the lipoidoses and usually showing a recessive, familial character, often commences before or at puberty. It is more slowly progressive than the infantile type. Symptoms usually start with a progressive loss of vision, later followed by mental deterioration and neurological symptoms in the form of progressive dementia and apathy, epileptiform attacks, ataxy, rigidity, and tremor. The electroretinographic response is extinguished already in the early stage. Death usually occurs about the age of 18 years.

OPHTHALMOSCOPICALLY, the fundus lesion is seen in the early stage as a small white spot in the fovea, while the optic disc and the retinal vessels are normal. The white spot is subsequently transformed into a larger pigmented spot, which is usually surrounded by a red halo (Fig. 310). As the disease progresses, the disc becomes pale and atrophic (Fig. 311), the retinal vessels narrow (Fig. 312), and the macular lesions increase in size.

Depigmentation and fine pigmentations are seen in both maculae (Fig. 312) and in the periphery (Fig. 313) of the fundi. At times, a number of fine whitish branching streaks radiate from the macula, but cherry-red spots or whitish zones in the maculae, as seen in the infantile type, do not occur.

The condition is easily distinguished from heredomacular degeneration and central choroiditis by the electroretinographic response, which is subnormal or extinguished in the juvenile form of amaurotic idiocy.

HISTOPATHOLOGICALLY, the retinal lesions are characterized by degeneration of the rods and cones and the pigment epithelium, simultaneous lipoidal degeneration of the ganglion cells, and glial proliferation.

In the central nervous system the changes are of the same type as in the infantile form, but in the juvenile type the affection is milder and unevenly distributed.

In the juvenile type of amaurotic family idiocy, vacuolated lymphocytes may occur as in Niemann-Pick's disease and in different acute infective conditions. Vacuolated lymphocytes, however, are not present in the infantile form of amaurotic family idiocy.

# Heredomacular Degeneration
### (Figures 314—325)

Heredomacular degeneration is a slowly progressive, often bilateral, degenerative condition affecting the macula. Although cases may occur without any family history, there is usually a strong family incidence, and the inheritance is

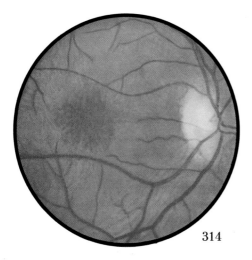

314

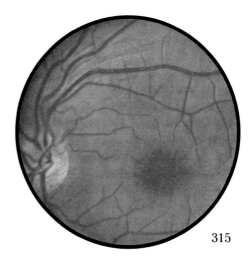

315

*Right eye. Heredomacular degeneration, early stage.*

*Left eye. Heredomacular degeneration, early stage.*

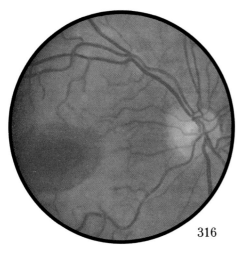

316

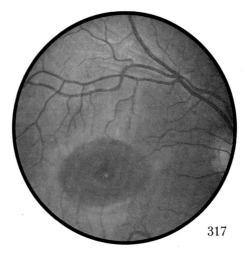

317

*Figures 316—319. Same right eye. The development of heredomacular degeneration. Figures*

*316 and 317 taken at 18 months' interval. Small white dot in the macula enlarged.*

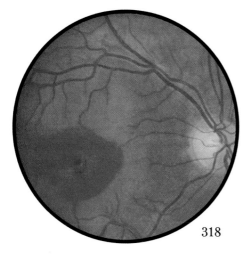

318

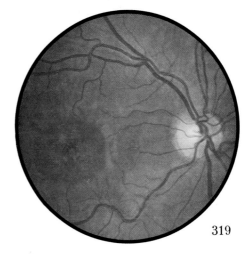

319

*Figures 318 and 319, ten months and 6 years later, show a further progression of the macular*

*degeneration. Disc and retinal vessels are normal.*

most frequently recessive.

Heredomacular degeneration may start at any age. According to the age of onset, the condition can be grouped into the following types: infantile (Best's type), juvenile (Stargardt's type), adult (Behr's type), presenile and senile. Most frequently, however, the condition appears in childhood or at puberty.

The principle complaint is a gradual, usually bilateral diminution of central vision. There is a relative or absolute central scotoma, the extent of which depends on the size of the macular lesion. The peripheral visual field is intact and the electroretinogram is normal. There are, however, no general symptoms.

OPHTHALMOSCOPICALLY, the infantile type commences as a vitelliform disc or cyst which is indistinguishable from a congenital vitelline macular cyst (Figs. 28—29). The evolution of the lesion is exceedingly slow. Finally, the lesion is converted into an atrophic scar with or without pigmentation.

OPHTHALMOSCOPICALLY, in the juvenile and adult type, the macular changes commence with a slight irregularity in pigmentation and are followed by some depigmentation and fine clumping of pigment.

At the early stage, a small whitish spot is frequently present in the fovea (Figs. 316—317), surrounded by a red halo, and fine whitish branching lines may radiate from the fovea (Figs. 314—315). This small whitish spot later disappears. Fully developed (Figs. 318—325), the macular degeneration is seen as a sharply demarcated, round or oval, reddish-brown or deep-red, often worm-eaten area measuring from one half to two disc diameters. Varying amounts of fine and coarse pigment deposits and depigmentations are situated in the macular lesion. Finally, the lesion may sometimes be surrounded by whitish patches resembling those seen in fundus flavimaculatus (Figs. 324—325).

The foveal reflex is absent from the onset, and the macular reflex disappears later. Occasionally, fine pigment accumulations are seen in the fundus periphery, but elsewhere the fundi appear normal. The optic discs and retinal vessels are normal.

The condition is in the early stage distinguished from the juvenile form of amaurotic family idiocy by the lack of electroretinographic changes, and later by differences in the ophthalmoscopic picture and a lack of general symptoms. The condition must not be confused with central choroiditis.

In the presenile and senile type, the macular lesions closely resemble those seen in senile macular degeneration.

HISTOPATHOLOGICALLY, there is degeneration of the neuroepithelium in the affected area, and degeneration and some proliferation of the retinal pigment epithelium.

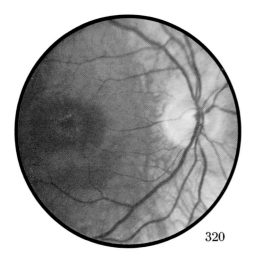

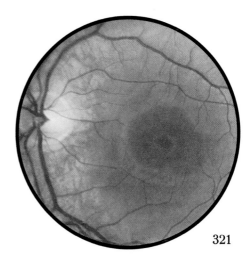

320

321

*Figures 320 and 321. Right and left eyes. Heredomacular degeneration. In both macular* areas there is a dark-red spot surrounded by a small atrophic zone.

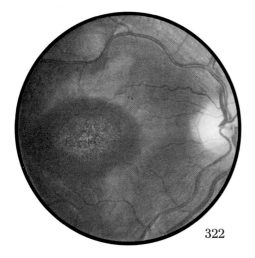

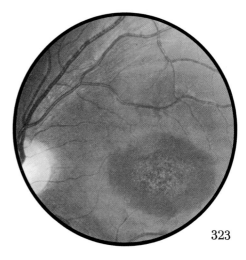

322

323

*Figures 322 and 323. Right and left eyes. Heredomacular degeneration, advanced stage. In* both macular areas there is an oval, worm-eaten, degenerative zone.

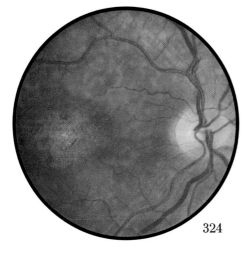

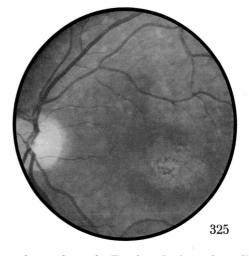

324

325

*Figures 324 and 325. Same eyes as figures 322 and 323, five years later. The macular lesions are* nearly unchanged. Fundus flavimaculatus-like, irregular light patches developed.

# Toxic Macular Degeneration

(Figures 326—331)

Toxic macular degeneration with pigmentary changes may be the result of various toxic substances or drugs, particularly tranquilizers such as chlorpromazine and thioridazine, and antimalarials such as chloroquine and its derivatives.

Visual disturbances may occur together with central, pericentral or paracentral scotomas, and the visual field may show concentric contraction.

OPHTHALMOSCOPICALLY, the macular area shows in the early stage a fine diffuse mottling, pigment clumping, depigmentation (Figs. 328—329) or a small hemorrhage. The condition is sometimes associated with slight edema in the adjacent area (Figs. 330—331). Later, a pale ring may surround the fovea to form a ring-shaped lesion (Figs. 326—327) called "bull's eye", or the lesion shows some pigment clumping. Pigmentary changes may also develop in the periphery. The retinal vessels may show a varying degree of contraction, and finally the optic disc may become atrophic.

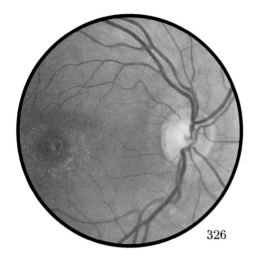

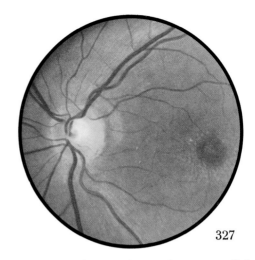

Figures 326 and 327. Right and left eyes. Toxic retinopathy (chloroquine). Both maculae show fine depigmentation and some small hard exudates.

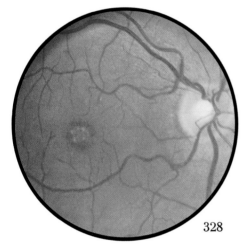

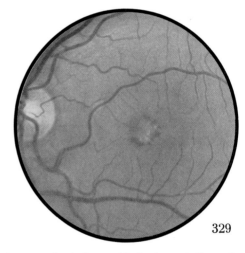

Figures 328 and 329. Right and left eyes. Toxic retinopathy (Mellaril). Both maculae show degenerative lesions with depigmentation, pigment clumping and small hemorrhages.

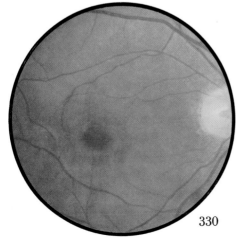

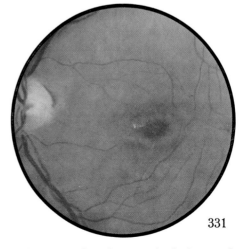

Figures 330 and 331. Right and left eyes. Toxic retinopathy (antimalarial drugs). Both macular areas show degenerative lesions and some edema.

# Senile Macular Degeneration
(Figures 332—341)

Senile macular degeneration is a condition resulting from vascular sclerosis, and it may often be closely related to senile disciform macular degeneration. At times, the process starts as senile macular degeneration and ends as disciform degeneration. Sometimes the former is seen in one eye and the latter in the other eye. Bilateral occurrence is frequent, although the degree of involvement may differ in the two eyes.

Senile macular degeneration occurs most frequently in the sixties and later.

Frequently, there is no correlation between the apparent extent of the fundus lesions and the degree of the visual disturbances. Central vision may either be normal or severely reduced, and reduction of vision may commence slowly or develop within a few days. Once developed, the visual disturbances are permanent.

OPHTHALMOSCOPICALLY, senile macular degeneration is seen at the early stage as fine pigment accumulation and depigmentation in the macular area (Figs. 332—333). In the course of months or years, the depigmented atrophic spots become enlarged and there may be a varying amount of pigment accumulation (Figs. 334—336). Frequently, the condition is accompanied by few or numerous, small or large colloid bodies (Figs. 337—341) in and around the macular area. In the latter case, the condition closely resembles the fundus lesion described as Doyne's honeycomb choroiditis or dystrophy.

The retinal vessels show a varying degree of sclerosis. The optic disc is normal and retinal hemorrhages are not characteristic.

HISTOPATHOLOGICALLY, the macular changes are characterized by depigmentation and atrophy of the retinal pigment cells, isolated pigment cell proliferation and degenerative changes in the layers of rods and cones. There are degenerative changes in Bruch's membrane, often associated with colloid bodies, and sclerosis and some atrophy of the choroidal vessels in the macular area.

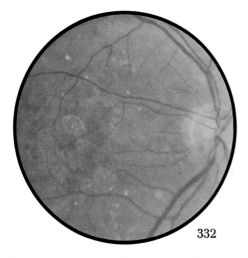

332

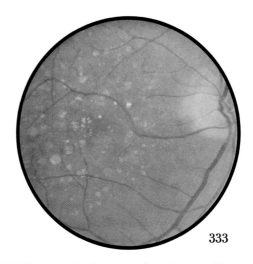

333

*Right eye. Senile macular degeneration. Some pigmentation and depigmentation in the macula.*

*Right eye. Senile macular degeneration and colloid bodies.*

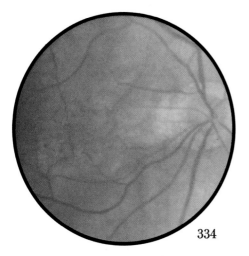

334

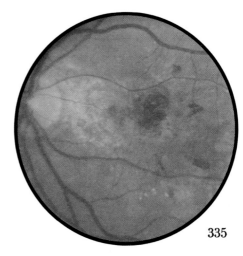

335

*Right eye. Senile macular degeneration with pigment clumping.*

*Left eye. Senile macular degeneration with coarse pigmentation.*

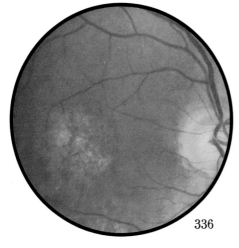

336

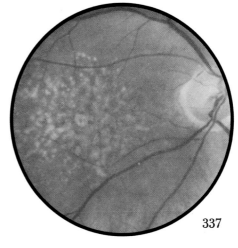

337

*Right eye. Senile macular degeneration with coarse depigmentation.*

*Right eye. Senile macular degeneration surrounded by colloid bodies.*

# Cystoid Degeneration of the Macula
(Figures 342—343)

Cystoid degeneration of the macula, just as cystoid degeneration in the fundal periphery, is due to a degenerative process with formation of small cystic cavities in the internuclear layer of the retina.

The condition occurs most often in old people, and visual disturbances may vary widely, from practically no complaints to the occurrence of a central scotoma.

OPHTHALMOSCOPICALLY, the lesion may be difficult to recognize in the early stage where small irregular reflexes may be the only sign of the condition. Later, however, the degeneration gives the macula a honeycombed appearance. Finally, a larger cystic cavity (Fig. 342) may be formed in the macula by coalescence of the small cystic spaces. If the anterior wall of this cystic cavity ruptures, it gives rise to a lamellar macular hole (Fig. 343). The distinction between a cystic cavity and a hole may be difficult in ordinary ophthalmoscopy, but is easily distinguished by using a slit-lamp together with a Hruby lens. The retinal vessels show a varying degree of sclerosis, and the optic disc is normal.

In cystoid macular degeneration, a lamellar macular hole very seldom gives rise to retinal detachment.

HISTOPATHOLOGICALLY, the condition is seen as cystoid spaces especially in the internuclear retinal layer, and is associated with some retinal degeneration. At times, the fovea presents a large cystic cavity or even a lamellar retinal hole. The underlying choroid usually shows sclerotic changes.

# Primary Choroidal Atrophy
(Figures 344—349)

Primary choroidal atrophy is a degenerative condition showing a heredofamilial tendency and characterized by choroidal atrophy and degenerative changes in the retina. The condition can be divided into three separate entities, central areolar choroidal atrophy, peripapillary choroidal atrophy and diffuse choroidal atrophy.

*Central areolar choroidal atrophy*
(Figs. 344—347).

Central areolar choroidal atrophy, which is usually bilateral, occurs most

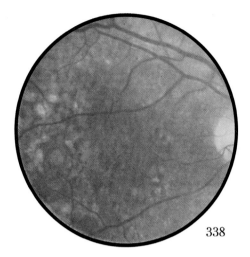

338

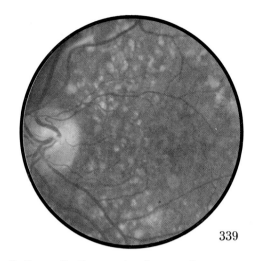

339

*Right eye. Senile macular degeneration surround-*
*ed by colloid bodies.*

*Left eye. Senile macular degeneration surrounded*
*by colloid bodies*

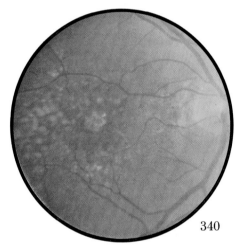

340

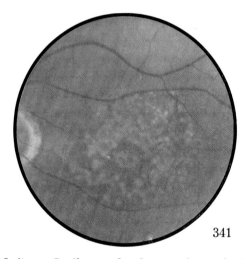

341

*Right eye. Senile macular degeneration surround-*
*ed by colloid bodies.*

*Left eye. Senile macular degeneration and colloid*
*bodies.*

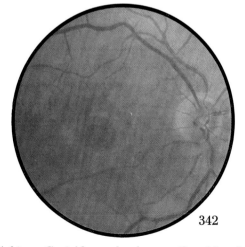

342

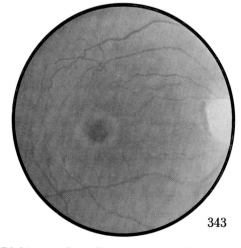

343

*Right eye. Cystoid macular degeneration. Macular*
*cyst seen as deep-red spot.*

*Right eye. Lamellar macular hole in cystoid*
*macular degeneration.*

frequently in middle-aged or older persons, but may already become evident at ages between 20 and 40 years.

Central vision may be severely reduced in early stages. However, central vision is often only slightly impaired in the early stage, but shows progressive diminution. When central vision is decreased, there is a central scotoma of varying extension but the peripheral field is intact.

OPHTHALMOSCOPICALLY, the early lesion is seen in the macular area as an ill-defined, sometimes irregular patch with retinal pigment atrophy and exposure of the choroidal vessels (Figs. 344—345). Sometimes slight edema and small hemorrhages may also be present. The fully developed macular lesion (Figs. 346—347) is well-defined, oval or round, measuring from one to four disc diameters. The affected area is whitish or yellowish-white due to choroidal atrophy. The choroidal vessels are diminished in number and the remaining vessels are sclerosed. Retinal pigment is nearly absent in the affected area.

### Peripapillary choroidal atrophy
(Fig. 348).

Peripapillary choroidal atrophy usually occurs in middle-aged or older persons.

The fundal lesion produces a visual field defect, and if the macula is also involved there is a central scotoma, but the peripheral field remains intact.

OPHTHALMOSCOPICALLY, the lesion (Fig. 348) is seen as an ill-defined area with exposure of the atrophic choroid and sclerosed choroidal vessels, together with some pigment clumping. At first, the lesion is located around the optic disc, but later it may also involve the macular area.

### Diffuse choroidal atrophy
(Fig. 349).

Diffuse choroidal atrophy usually occurs in middle-aged persons, but is not infrequently seen already in the thirties.

Visual symptoms may be absent in the early stages, while later the visual fields usually show a progressive contraction. If the macular area is involved, central vision is markedly reduced. Night blindness is often present and the electroretinographic response is subnormal or even extinguished.

OPHTHALMOSCOPICALLY, there is a more or less diffuse exposure of the choroidal vessels (Fig. 349), seen as a network of grayish or grayish-white lines, and between these lines the fundus has assumed a grayish or grayish-brown color. Small or large irregular masses of pigment clumping are often present in the equatorial region. The optic disc and the retinal vessels usually appear normal.

Primary choroidal atrophy should not be confused with choroideremia or gyrate choroidal atrophy.

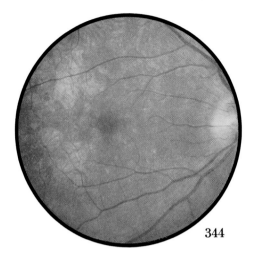

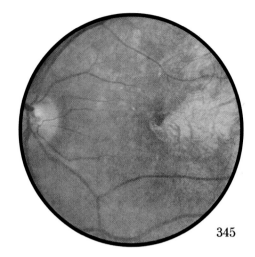

*Figures 344 and 345. Right and left eyes. Central areolar choroidal atrophy, early stages.*   *The discs and retinal vessels are normal.*

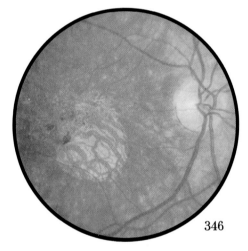

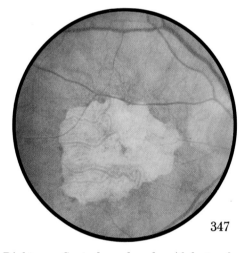

*Right eye. Central areolar choroidal atrophy.*   *Right eye. Central areolar choroidal atrophy and sclerosis of choroidal vessels.*

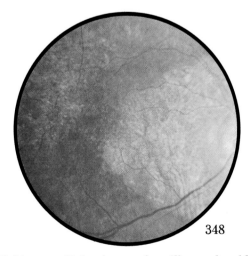

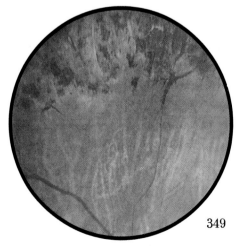

*Right eye. Extensive peripapillary choroidal atrophy.*   *Right eye. Diffuse choroidal atrophy with marked pigmentation.*

# Juvenile Disciform Degeneration
# of the Macula
### (Figures 350—361)

Juvenile disciform macular degeneration most frequently affects individuals in the twenties. The ophthalmoscopic appearance is very much like the senile form of disciform macular degeneration, but in the juvenile group there is no evidence of vascular disease. The condition becomes bilateral in about 50 per cent of the cases.

The visual complaints vary considerably depending on the localization and extension of the fundal lesion. In the early stage, the patients most often complain of metamorphopsia and blurring of vision. In some cases a permanent central scotoma may develop, in others a paracentral scotoma develops and central vision remains normal or becomes slightly reduced. The peripheral visual field remains intact.

OPHTHALMOSCOPICALLY, the fundus lesion may start in one of two ways. In the one, it starts as a small indistinct edematous, grayish or yellowish-white fleck in the central part of the macula (Figs. 359—360) or perifoveally in the macular area (Figs. 356—357). The fleck, which soon enlarges, seldom becomes larger than two disc diameters. Small subretinal hemorrhages may often border the lesion. In the other process, fundus changes start with a rounded, dark-red or slate-gray subretinal hemorrhage of about disc size (Figs. 350—353). The hemorrhage is gradually absorbed, leaving a grayish or yellowish-white area.

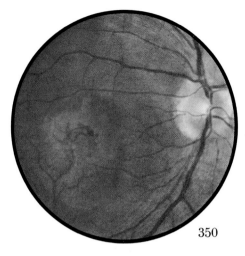

350

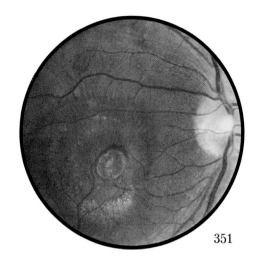

351

*Figures 350—355. Same right eye. The pic-*
*tures show the development of a juvenile disci-*

*form macular degeneration in the course of*
*17 months. The lesion commences with a macular*

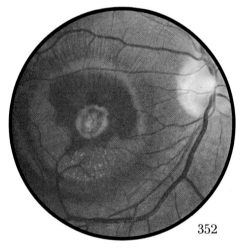

352

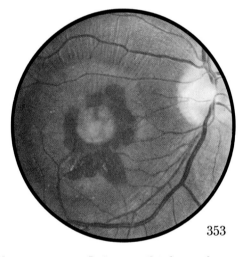

353

*subretinal hemorrhage and some edema. In*
*the further development a new subretinal hemor-*

*rhage appears. Later on the hemorrhages are*
*absorbed and the lesion converted into a fibrous*

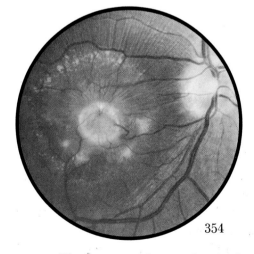

354

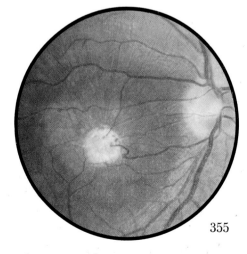

355

*tissue scar. Finally, some pigmentation develops*
*at the margin of the scar. Disc and retinal*

*vessels are normal.*

In nearly all cases, a final fibrotic stage is reached, which is the same in both processes described. At this stage (Figs. 354—355, 358), the lesion is seen as a rounded, whitish or yellowish-white, slightly elevated mass, measuring from one to two disc diameters. The fibrotic mass may be surrounded by small glistening white exudates (Fig. 354). Occasionally, the final stage shows a more diffuse chorioretinal scarring (Fig. 361). The retinal vessels and the optic disc appear normal.

In the early stage, the condition may be confused with a commencing malignant choroidal melanoma and an acute choroiditis, but the conditions may be distinguished by fluorescein angiography, as they usually show different patterns of fluorescence. Clinically they are soon distinguished, as their course differs.

HISTOPATHOLOGICALLY, the changes resemble those of the senile type of disciform macular degeneration, but the choroid shows no evidence of vascular disease.

# Senile Disciform Degeneration of the Macula
(Figures 362—371)

Senile disciform macular degeneration most frequently affects individuals over the age of 60 years. The condition is closely related to vascular sclerosis and often to senile macular degeneration. At times, senile macular degeneration is found in one eye and disciform degeneration in the other. The condition becomes bilateral in about 50 per cent of the cases.

The patients complain of suddenly occurring metamorphopsia and blurred vision, which is soon followed by a permanent central scotoma. The peripheral visual field, however, remains intact.

OPHTHALMOSCOPICALLY, the fundus lesion may start in one of two different ways. In the one, it starts as a small, slightly elevated, grayish-red or yellowish, often edematous indistinct fleck in the macula (Figs. 362, 364, 368—369). The fleck soon enlarges, and gradually involves the whole macular area. During progression, subretinal hemorrhages often border the lesion (Fig. 368). In the other process, fundus changes (Figs. 366, 370) start with a rounded, irregular, dark-red, grayish-green or greenish subretinal hemorrhage, which is gradually absorbed, leaving a grayish or yellowish-white area.

Finally, a fibrotic stage is reached, which is the same in both processes described (Figs. 363, 365, 367, 371). In this

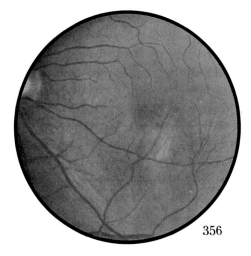

356

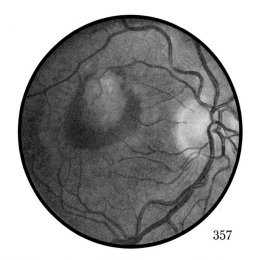

357

*Left eye. Juvenile disciform macular degeneration, early stage.*

*Right eye. Juvenile disciform macular degeneration, early stage.*

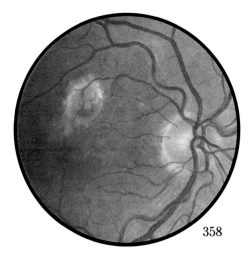

358

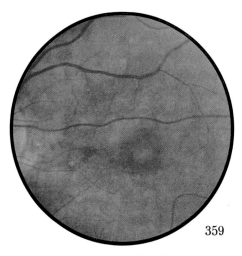

359

*Same eye as figure 357, fifteen months later. Chorioretinal scar.*

*Left eye. Incipient juvenile disciform macular degeneration.*

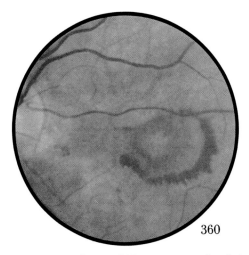

360

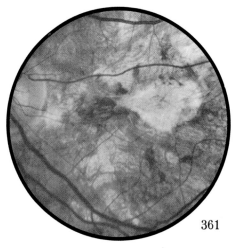

361

*Same eye as figure 359, two months later. Macular lesion progressing.*

*Same eye as figure 360, six years later. Disciform chorioretinal scar.*

stage, there is a rounded, grayish or yel-lowish-white mass in the macular area, measuring from a few to several disc dia-meters, and often projecting forward for several diopters. Not infrequently, the central mass is surrounded by glistening white exudates arranged in a circinate manner (Fig. 365). The retinal vessels may show a varying degree of sclerosis. The disc, however, is normal.

In the early stage, senile disciform macular degeneration may be confused with a commencing malignant choroidal melanoma and an acute choroiditis, but the conditions may be distinguished by fluorescein angiography, as they usually show different patterns of fluorescence. Clinically they are soon distinguished, as their course differs.

HISTOPATHOLOGICALLY, the lesions are largely confined to the macular area. In the early stage, fresh blood or albuminous exudate is accumulated beneath the reti-nal pigment epithelium, between the pig-ment epithelium and the neuroepithe-lium, and in the subretinal area. Ruptures are found in Bruch's membrane and the retinal layers are pushed forward by the blood or exudate. Later, the process be-comes organized, the retinal pigment epi-thelium proliferates, and new-formed vessels and connective tissue cells extend from the choroid into the exudate or blood. Finally, the retina is elevated by a dense layer of relatively avascular connective tissue. The outer retinal ele-ments show complete degeneration, leav-ing cystic spaces, and the inner layers show marked atrophy. In the macular area there is also marked sclerosis and atrophy of the choroidal vessels.

# Circinate Retinopathy
## (Figures 372—373)

Circinate retinopathy or retinitis cir-cinata is a relatively uncommon condition characterized by a girdle of exudates sur-rounding the macular area. In the ma-jority of cases, the condition is seen in elderly persons showing evidence of se-nile vascular disease, and is often asso-ciated with conditions such as senile ma-cular degeneration or senile disciform macular degeneration. Circinate retino-pathy, however, may also occur in other conditions with disturbances of the fun-dal circulation, especially diabetic retino-pathy, venous occlusion and sometimes in Coats' syndrome or angiomatosis of the retina.

Visual disturbances depend on the de-gree of macular involvement, but cen-tral vision usually becomes gradually di-minished and a central scotoma develops. The peripheral visual field, however, is left intact.

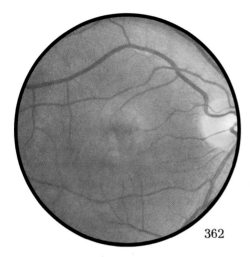

362

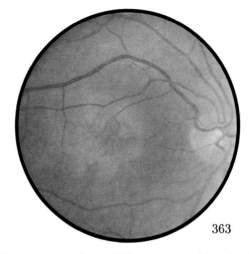

363

*Right eye. Incipient senile disciform macular degeneration.*

*Same eye as figure 362, six years later. Lesion enlarged somewhat.*

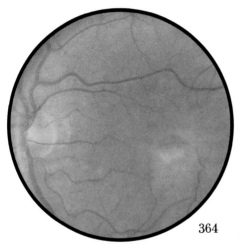

364

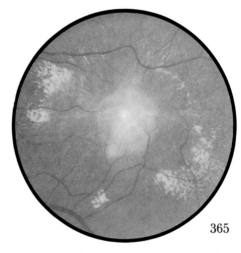

365

*Left eye. Senile disciform macular degeneration, early stage.*

*Same eye as figure 364, six months later. Scar stage with hard exudates.*

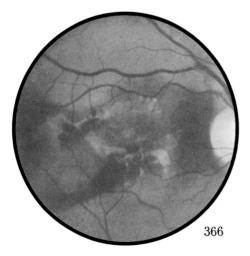

366

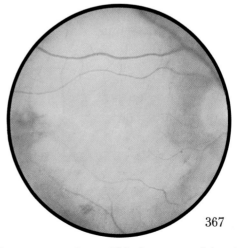

367

*Right eye. Senile disciform macular degeneration, early stage.*

*Same eye as figure 366, four years later. Scar stage.*

In senile cases the condition is frequently bilateral, although the eyes may be unequally affected or the development in the second eye may be delayed for some years.

OPHTHALMOSCOPICALLY, circinate retinopathy (Figs. 372—373) is seen as a complete or incomplete girdle of sharply defined, deep, discrete or confluent, glistening white or yellowish-white exudates surrounding the macular area. The lesion is usually bound by the upper and lower temporal retinal vessels. The macular area frequently shows degenerative changes (Fig. 373) resembling those seen in senile macular degeneration or senile disciform macular degeneration. In advanced cases, the exudates may also involve the macula, and small retinal hemorrhages may occur among the exudates. The condition usually shows a steady progression, but in some cases the exudates may be absorbed again, leaving only small pigmentary changes while the macular lesion remains. The retinal vessels show some sclerosis and the optic disc is usually normal.

HISTOPATHOLOGICALLY, the condition is characterized by an accumulation of fat-filled phagocytes in the middle and outer retinal layers, interspersed by free masses of lipid material. The adjacent retinal elements show a varying degree of degeneration. The area enclosed by the exudates shows varying degrees of cystoid, senile or disciform degeneration.

# Colloid Bodies (Drusen)
(Figures 333, 337—341 and 374—376)

Colloid bodies, also known as hyaline bodies or drusen, are mound-like excrescences in Bruch's membrane. Their nature is not quite clear. Colloid bodies may occur in otherwise normally appearing fundi (Figs. 374, 376), they may be present as a senile phenomenon (Figs. 333, 337—341, 375) or as a degenerative phenomenon in vascular, inflammatory or neoplastic fundal conditions.

A certain condition presenting an accumulation of colloid bodies in the macular area, and occurring as a heredo-familial disease, initially without visual symptoms but eventually showing some degree of macular degeneration is known as Doyne's honeycomb choroiditis or dystrophy.

Colloid bodies may be seen at all ages, but occur most frequently in individuals over 60 years. In themselves, they do not cause any visual disturbances.

OPHTHALMOSCOPICALLY, they are seen as yellowish or yellowish-white pinpoint dots or larger rounded spots situated beneath the retinal vessels (Figs. 374—376). They may be few in number or numerous, scattered anywhere in the fun-

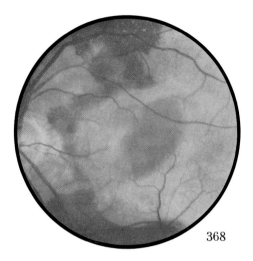

368

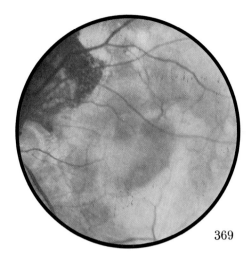

369

*Left eye. Senile disciform macular degeneration, early stage.*

*Same eye as figure 368, nine months later. Scarring stage.*

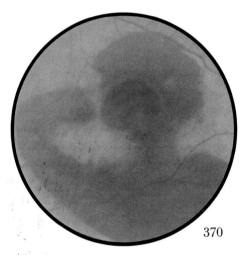

370

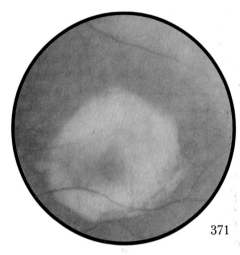

371

*Left eye. Senile disciform macular degeneration, early stage.*

*Same eye as figure 370, eight months later. Hemorrhage replaced by scar.*

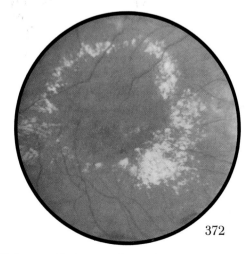

372

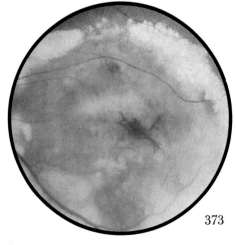

373

*Right eye. Circinate retinopathy, early stage.*

*Left eye. Circinate retinopathy with advanced macular degeneration.*

dus, and often form large aggregates, especially in the macular area and around the disc. When large, they may be slightly elevated. At times, the single lesion is bordered by slight pigmentation.

HISTOPATHOLOGICALLY, the membrane of Bruch is thickened and shows flat, round or mound-like PAS-positive projections. In early stages, the projections are covered by retinal pigment epithelium, but when the excrescences enlarge the pigment epithelium becomes flattened, depigmented or disappears entirely at the site of the excrescences.

# Central Serous Retinopathy
### (Figures 377—378)

The etiology of central serous retinopathy is unknown, but several theories have been advanced, including vasomotor instability and allergy. The term central serous retinopathy is applied to different conditions, all presenting a well-defined edema in the macular area and clinically behaving in the same way, even if in some cases the edema is located in the retina and in others is located preretinally or subretinally.

The condition is usually unilateral and affects most often young or middle-aged males.

The patient complains of hazy vision, metamorphopsia, micropsia, positive central or paracentral scotoma, and objects may appear as if seen through sun-glasses. In most cases, there is complete recovery of vision in the course of weeks or some months. However, recurrences are common and may occasionally lead to permanent impairment of vision.

OPHTHALMOSCOPICALLY, central serous retinopathy is seen as a slightly elevated zone of indistinctness in the macular area, measuring from one to two disc diameters (Figs. 377—378). The involved area resembles a flat vesicle and is sharply outlined by a circular or oval light reflex. The color is grayish-red or deeper red than normal, and the retinal vessels in the affected area are slightly tortuous and contracted. Small white dots are frequently present within the affected area (Fig. 378). The condition may subside, leaving a normal macular area or one with some atrophy and pigment disturbances, or even cystoid degeneration, eventually followed by a lamellar macular hole.

Central serous retinopathy is relatively often associated with an optic pit or hole in the temporal part of the optic disc (Fig. 377).

In ordinary ophthalmoscopy it is usually impossible to determine whether the edema is preretinal, retinal or subretinal. Using a slit-lamp together with a Hruby lens, however, it is easy to determine the position of the serous fluid.

HISTOPATHOLOGICALLY, there is a preretinal, retinal or subretinal accumulation of serous fluid together with some degenerative changes in the retina in the foveal region.

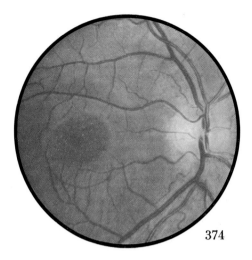

374

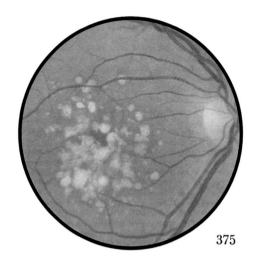

375

*Right eye. Accumulation of small drusen (colloid bodies) in the macular area.*

*Right eye. Large colloid bodies in the macular area.*

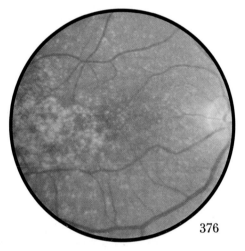

376

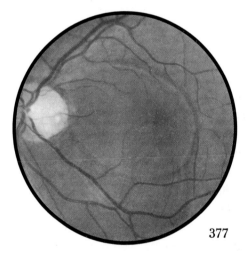

377

*Right eye. The fundus is speckled with pinpoint drusen (colloid bodies).*

*Left eye. Central serous retinopathy and crater-like hole in the optic disc.*

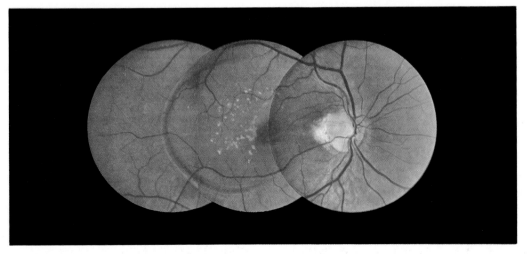

*Figure 378. Composite picture. Right eye. Central serous retinopathy, seen as a slightly prominent area of indistinctness in the macular area, bordered by a light reflex.*

# Coats' Syndrome
(Figures 379—384)

Coats' syndrome may be divided into two groups. The first is characterized from the very beginning by massive retinal and subretinal exudate, with or without gross vascular disease. The second, also called Leber's multiple miliary aneurysms, commences with retinal arterial aneurysms and only slight exudative changes. The exudates, however, usually progress, so that the late stages may be indistinguishable. The condition is probably always due to a vascular malformation, primarily affecting the retinal vessels in the diseased area of the fundus.

The syndrome occurs most frequently in apparently healthy young persons, especially males, and usually affects one eye only. In most cases the disease is slowly and steadily progressive, but may remain stationary for long periods.

In early stages there are no or only slight visual complaints. Later, vision may be reduced to a varying degree, depending on the localization and extension of the pathological process.

OPHTHALMOSCOPICALLY, the fundus changes in the first group are characterized (Figs. 379—383) by well-defined or soft-edged, yellowish or whitish, flat or prominent, single or confluent exudates situated beneath the retinal vessels. The exudates are usually localized near the optic disc (Fig. 379) or the macula (Fig. 382), but may also occur in the periphery (Fig. 381). Small retinal hemorrhages may be diffusely scattered in the fundus. Fusiform or spherical dilatations (Figs. 380—382) and tortuosities preferentially of the retinal arteries frequently occur at several sites. Occasionally, angioma-like lesions (Fig. 383) may also be present. Sheathing of the retinal vessels is common (Fig. 380). In the early stage, some vitreous haze may be present. In the late stages, the exudates may cover the whole fundus and finally retinitis proliferans and retinal detachment may develop.

In the second group the fundus changes (Fig. 384) commence with fusiform or spherical dilatations, arterial and sometimes also venous aneurysms, and tortuosities of the retinal vessels in different areas of the fundus. At first, there may be no exudates, only some sheathing of the diseased vessels or slight exudation around the diseased vessels. In the course of time, however, the exudates usually enlarge so that the late stages and final appearance may be indistinguishable from that described in the first group.

In the differential diagnosis, it is necessary to consider retinoblastoma, angiomatosis of the retina and posterior uveitis.

HISTOPATHOLOGICALLY, the early stages are characterized by a serofibrinous exudate involving all retinal layers. Necroses are often present in the outer retinal layers, and widely dilated and thin-walled capillary vessels are frequently found in the inner layers. An extensive exudate, invaded by characteristic large,

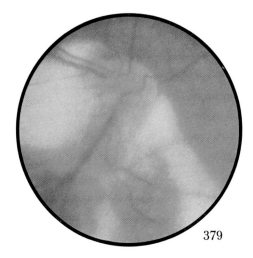

379

*Right eye. Coats' syndrome. Confluent, deeply situated whitish exudates.*

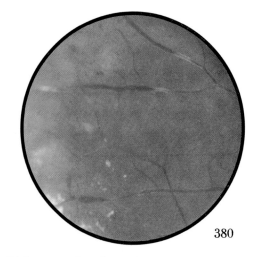

380

*Right eye. Coats' syndrome. Aneurysms and sheathing of retinal vessels.*

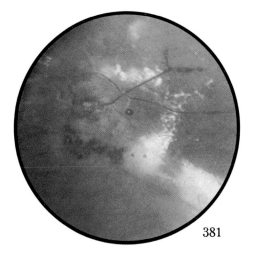

381

*Same eye as figure 380. Numerous miliary aneurysms and deep exudates.*

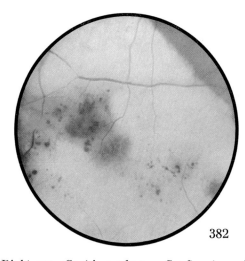

382

*Right eye. Coats' syndrome. Confluent exudate and microaneurysms.*

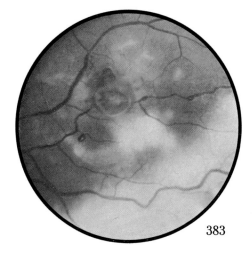

383

*Left eye. Coats' syndrome. Exudates, aneurysms and angiomatous tumor.*

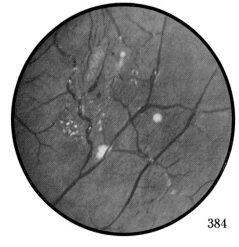

384

*Left eye. Coats' syndrome. Leber's multiple miliary aneurysms.*

pale-staining histiocytes, is formed between the retinal pigment epithelium and the main retina, which then becomes detached. Finally, the exudate is replaced by fibrous tissue deep in the retina or between the retina and the choroid.

# Angioid Streaks
(Figures 385—395)

Angioid streaks are a rare, slowly progressive degenerative condition characterized by ruptures in Bruch's membrane and frequently associated with macular degeneration.

Angioid streaks may occur with or without evidence of systemic disease. Most frequently the condition is found in association with pseudoxanthoma elasticum, which is an uncommon systemic disease, having a familial character and showing a heredity of the recessive type. It is characterized by a generalized degeneration of the elastic tissue of the body, mainly affecting the skin, ocular fundus and cardiovascular system. The complex of angioid streaks and pseudoxanthoma elasticum is known as the Grönblad-Strandberg syndrome. Occasionally, angioid streaks have been observed in Ehlers-Danlos' syndrome, Paget's disease and sickle-cell anemia.

Angioid streaks may occur at all ages. The condition is always bilateral, but the eyes are usually unequally affected.

In early stages, there are usually no visual complaints. In long-standing cases, however, the macula is usually involved and this may seriously affect the visual acuity. Finally, vision may be further impaired by visual field defects occurring in association with an extensive choroidal atrophy.

Angioid streaks are often associated with systemic diseases and especially with pseudoxanthoma elasticum, with wide-spread degeneration of the elastic tissue. In these cases the vascular changes may lead to serious disturbances of function in other systems, and the general prognosis is determined by the systemic disease.

Ophthalmoscopically, the angioid streaks are seen as fine or broad, brown, red or grayish wavy bands with tapering ends, situated beneath the retinal vessels (Figs. 385—387). They may resemble blood vessels and are often bordered by some pigment or a whitish line (Fig. 388). The angioid streaks frequently anastomose near the optic disc, forming an irregular ring around it, and then radiating towards the equatorial region. In the macular and perimacular area and sometimes also in the fundus periphery, coarse granulation may be present, giving rise to the so-called peau d'orange configuration (Figs. 387—388). In the fundus periphery, scattered, yellowish-white or whitish spots, known as salmon spots (Fig. 389), often associated with some pigment deposits resembling small chorioretinal scars or colloid bodies, are often present in long-standing cases. Small or large retinal or preretinal hemorrhages may also occur. Macular changes usually

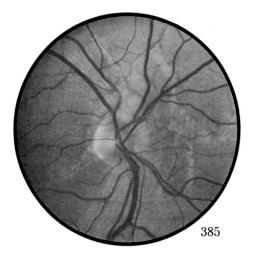

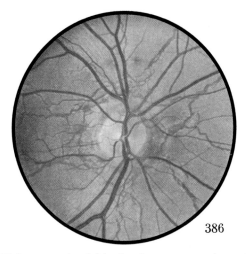

385

386

*Right eye. Angioid streaks, seen as irregular red-brown and grayish bands around the disc.*

*Right eye. Angioid streaks, seen as irregular red-brown anastomosing bands.*

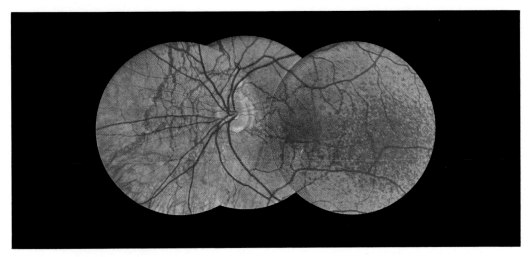

*Figure 387. Composite picture. Left eye. There are numerous angioid streaks nasally. In the*  *perimacular area the fundus has assumed a peau d'orange configuration.*

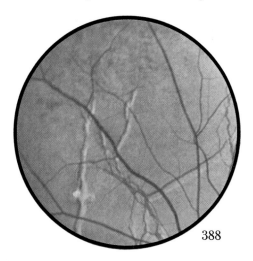

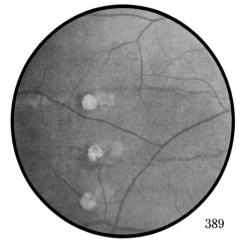

388

389

*Left eye. Angioid streaks accompanied by irregular whitish lines.*

*Right eye. Angioid streaks and yellowish-white "salmon"-spots.*

develop about the age of 50 years. The lesions resemble disciform macular degeneration (Figs. 390—394). Finally, patchy areas of choroidal sclerosis appear and become confluent. They form large, sharply defined lobulated zones of atrophy, with exposure of the choroidal vessels and pigment deposits (Fig. 395), and the angioid streaks disappear entirely in these atrophic areas.

Histopathologically, irregular defects and ruptures in Bruch's membrane are found at the site of the angioid streaks, and the breaks show jagged edges and vary in breadth. Connective tissue from the choroid may fill the defects and the pigment epithelium may show both hypertrophy and atrophy in association with the defects. In the advanced stage, disciform degeneration is found in the macula. The choriocapillaris may be atrophic and replaced by collagenous connective tissue.

# Retinal Perivasculitis
(Figures 396—397, 399—401, 403, 408, 410 and 412—413)

Retinal perivasculitis is an inflammatory condition including both periphlebitis and periarteritis. Most frequently the retinal veins are involved, more rarely the retinal arteries. Sometimes, however, both arteries and veins are affected.

Retinal perivasculitis may occur in conditions as for example Eales' disease, multiple sclerosis, uveitis and acute retinochoroiditis or in diseases such as tuberculosis and syphilis.

# Eales' Disease
(Figures 396—399)

Eales' disease is a condition of unknown etiology characterized by retinal periphlebitis and a tendency to recurrent vitreous hemorrhages.

As a rule, both eyes are affected, and in the early stages one more than the other.

The disease occurs most frequently in healthy young individuals, especially males. Occasionally there is a history of tuberculosis.

In the periphlebitic stage, there are no or only slight visual disturbances. The occurrence of vitreous hemorrhage, how-

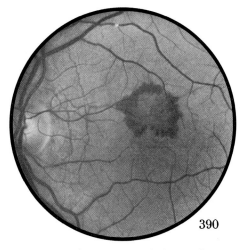

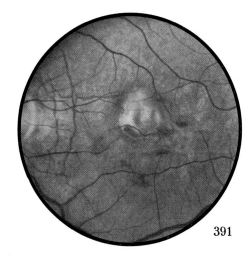

Left eye. Macular subretinal hemorrhage and angioid streaks.

Same eye as figure 390, nine months later. Chorioretinal macular scar.

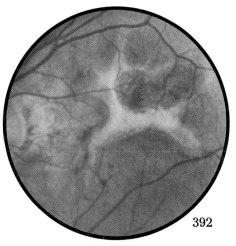

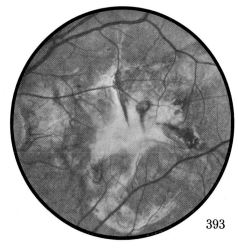

Left eye. Chorioretinal macular scar, early stage, and angioid streaks.

Same eye as figure 392, two years later. Firm fibrous tissue in the macula.

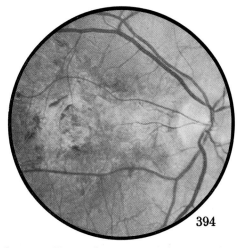

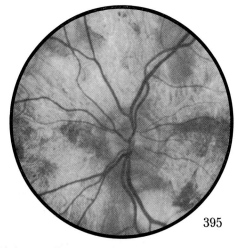

Right eye. From the same patient as figures 392 and 393. Chorioretinal macular scar.

Right eye. Extensive, heavy chorioretinal atrophy in angioid streaks.

ever, causes a blurring or loss of vision. Following the first few attacks the vitreous may clear again in the course of some weeks or months, but recurrent vitreous hemorrhages may develop after varying intervals, causing permanent damage with reduction of vision.

OPHTHALMOSCOPICALLY, the early stage is characterized by perivasculitic and mainly periphlebitic changes in different areas, especially towards the periphery (Figs. 396—397). Small retinal hemorrhages and chorioretinal foci are often present and small fan-shaped preretinal neovascularizations (Figs. 397—398) may occur in the periphery. The first vitreous hemorrhages may be absorbed and leave only some vitreous opacities. Recurrent hemorrhages, however, may be absorbed very slowly, often leading to retinitis proliferans (Figs. 398—399) with formation of new-formed vessels and connective tissue, preretinally and in the vitreous. The proliferative retinopathy may sooner or later cause traction on the retina, resulting in retinal detachment.

In the periphlebitic stage, the condition must be distinguished from periphlebitis in multiple sclerosis and in uveitis.

In the proliferative stage, it must be distinguished from proliferative diabetic retinopathy.

In the differential diagnosis of vitreous hemorrhage it is necessary to consider for example Eales' disease, angiomatosis of the retina, diabetic retinopathy, malignant choroidal melanoma and retinal detachment.

HISTOPATHOLOGICALLY, the retinal vessels and especially the veins show vasculitis and perivasculitis. The vessel walls are inflamed, their lumina sometimes occluded and they are often surrounded by lymphocytes. The late stages show retinitis proliferans and retinal detachment.

## Multiple Sclerosis
### (Figures 400—401)

Transient retinal periphlebitis is a frequent occurrence in the course of multiple sclerosis, in addition to retrobulbar neuritis, optic atrophy and eye muscle palsies. The periphlebitis, however, does not cause any visual disturbances.

OPHTHALMOSCOPICALLY, the periphlebitic changes are mainly found in the periphery of the fundus (Figs. 400—401). The veins are more or less obscured by whitish fluffy exudates which ensheath a single or several veins for a shorter or longer distance, and whitish plaques sometimes lie in front of the veins. The periphlebitic changes persist for some time and then disappear, but frequently new ones appear elsewhere. Occasionally, the retinal periphlebitis is associated with uveitis, but retinal hemorrhages and retinitis proliferans do not occur.

The condition must be distinguished from periphlebitis in Eales' disease and in uveitis.

HISTOPATHOLOGICALLY, the fundal lesions present a picture of retinal periphlebitis.

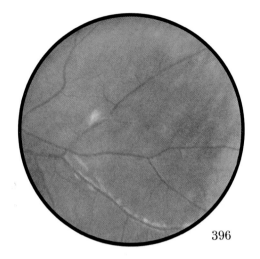

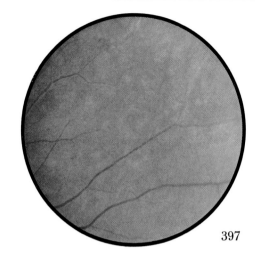

396

397

*Left eye. Periphlebitis in Eales' disease.*

*Right eye. Periphlebitis and neovascularization in Eales' disease.*

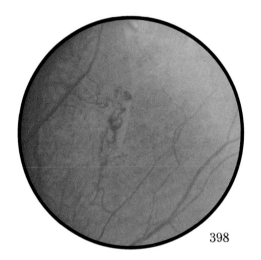

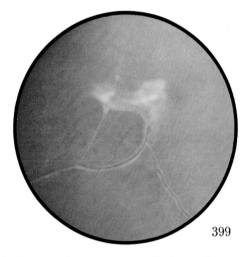

398

399

*Right eye. Neovascularization in Eales'disease.*

*Left eye. From same patient as figure 398. Sheathing and fibrous tissue.*

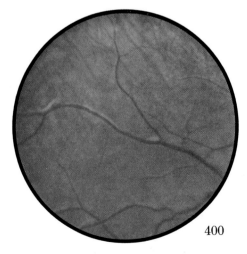

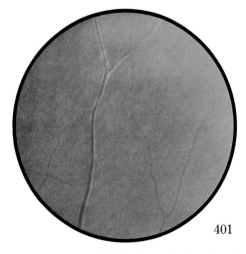

400

401

*Right eye. Periphlebitis in multiple sclerosis.*

*Right eye. Periphlebitis in multiple sclerosis.*

# Fundus Changes in Uveitis
(Figures 402—406 and 472)

Fundus changes in uveitis consist mainly of retinal edema and periphlebitis.

OPHTHALMOSCOPICALLY, the retinal edema in this condition may be localized to the macular area or widespread (Fig. 402), giving the retina a dull appearance with abnormal light reflexes. Occasionally, an exudative retinal detachment develops (Fig. 472). When the edema subsides, hard exudates may develop in the macular area (Figs. 404—405).

Retinal periphlebitis (Fig. 403) may occur with sheathing of the veins for a variable distance, and in sarcoidosis this sheathing is often associated with dense preretinal vitreous opacities (Fig. 406), which may remain unchanged after the uveitis and periphlebitis have subsided.

In the differential diagnosis, periphlebitic changes in Eales' disease and in multiple sclerosis have to be considered.

# Scintillatio Albescens and Synchysis Scintillans
(Figure 407)

Scintillatio albescens is a rare condition of unknown etiology. It usually affects individuals about the age of 60 years and is bilateral in about 75 per cent of the cases. Visual acuity is slightly reduced or normal.

OPHTHALMOSCOPICALLY, scintillatio albescens is seen as numerous small, round or disc-shaped, white, snowball-like vitreous opacities showing only slight movements when the eye is moved, and typically occurring in a vitreous which is otherwise of normal appearance.

HISTOPATHOLOGICAL AND HISTOCHEMICAL studies support the view that these vitreous opacities consist chiefly of calcium soaps.

Synchysis scintillans occurs most often in young adults and is frequently bilateral. The condition is often the consequence of other ocular diseases such as chronic degeneration, trauma, hemorrhage or inflammation.

OPHTHALMOSCOPICALLY, synchysis scintillans (Fig. 407) is seen as innumerable freely movable, glistening flakes in a fluid vitreous, often reflecting the ophthalmoscopic light with a golden sheen.

HISTOPATHOLOGICALLY AND HISTOCHEMICALLY, the opacities consist chiefly of crystalline deposits of cholesterol.

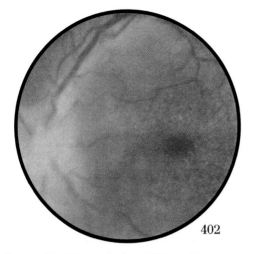

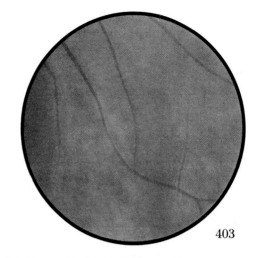

402

403

Left eye. Uveitis and choroiditis with macular edema.

Right eye. Periphlebitis in uveitis.

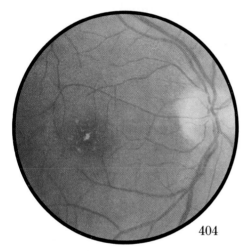

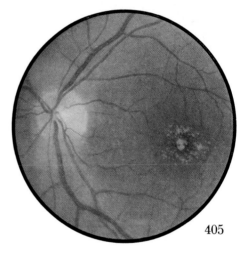

404

405

Figures 404 and 405. Right and left eyes. Sequelae after uveitis. Both maculae present hard

exudates following an inflammatory retinal edema.

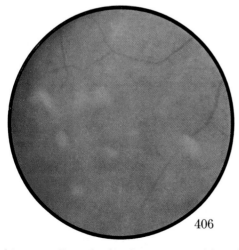

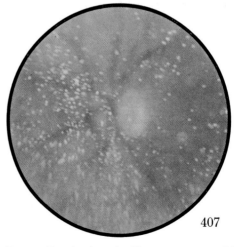

406

407

Right eye. Preretinal vitreous opacities in sarcoidosis.

Left eye. Synchysis scintillans, seen as whitish vitreous opacities.

# Retinal Arteritis and Periarteritis

(Figures 408—413)

Retinal arteritis and periarteritis may occur as the only manifestation of retinal vasculitis. More frequently, however, the condition is seen in association with retinal periphlebitis.

OPHTHALMOSCOPICALLY, numerous whitish patches border and partially cover the retinal arteries from the disc and a variable distance into the fundus (Fig. 408). The arteritis may subside leaving no trace, or giving rise to some constriction of the retinal arteries (Fig. 409) or even the formation of an arterial occlusion.

Sometimes, retinal arteritis is observed in association with acute chorioretinitis (Figs. 410—413).

In uveitis and Eales' disease, periarteritic changes may be present together with periphlebitic changes in the fundus periphery.

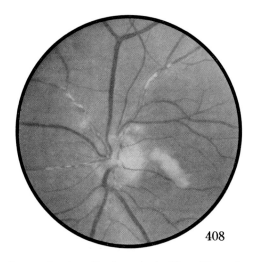

408

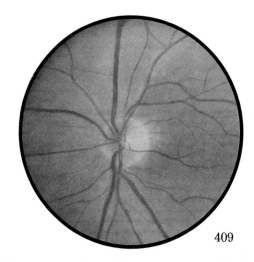

409

*Left eye. Acute retinal periarteritis with ensheathing and fluffy exudates.*

*Same eye as figure 408, one year later. Exudates and sheathing disappeared.*

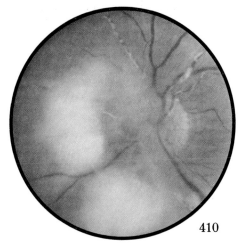

410

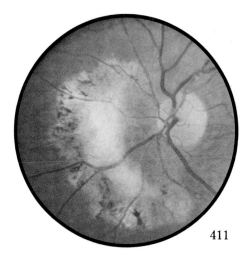

411

*Left eye. Posterior uveitis and retinal periarteritis, acute stage.*

*Same eye as figure 410, three years later. Scar stage.*

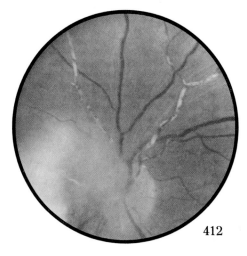

412

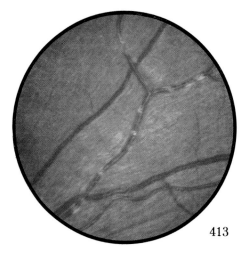

413

*Left eye. Posterior uveitis and retinal periarteritis, acute stage.*

*Same eye as figure 412, three years later (15°). Still some sheathing.*

# Choroiditis
(Figures 414—436)

Choroiditis or posterior uveitis is an inflammatory condition usually starting in the choroid and subsequently involving the retina. Sometimes, however, it may be secondary to retinitis and anterior uveitis.

Choroiditis is most frequently a non-suppurative inflammation of endogenous origin, caused by bacterial, viral, mycotic or parasitic agents, or very often a reaction due to toxic or allergic insults.

Choroiditis may occur in conditions such as tuberculosis, congenital syphilis, the secondary and tertiary stages of acquired syphilis, congenital or acquired toxoplasmosis, brucellosis, prenatal rubella infection, sarcoidosis, etc. In the vast majority of cases, however, the etiology is difficult or impossible to determine clinically in spite of extensive examination, including serological tests.

Choroiditis may occur at any age and is frequently bilateral. It may start insidiously, with no or only slight visual disturbances, or may be acute with hazy vision, metamorphopsia, macropsia, mi-

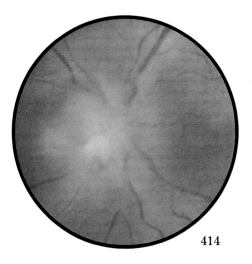

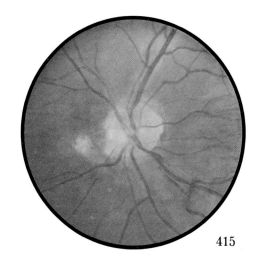

414

415

*Left eye. Juxtapapillary choroiditis in toxoplasmosis, acute stage.*

*Same eye as figure 414, six years later. Juxtapapillary choroiditis, scar stage.*

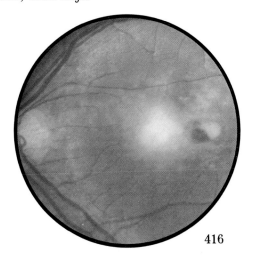

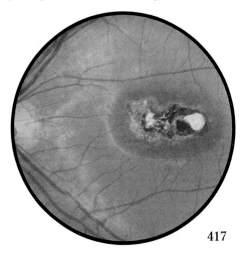

416

417

*Left eye. Central choroiditis of unknown origin, acute stage. Chorioretinal scar also present.*

*Same eye as figure 416, two years later. Central choroiditis, scar stage.*

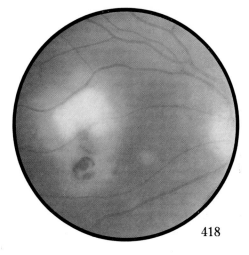

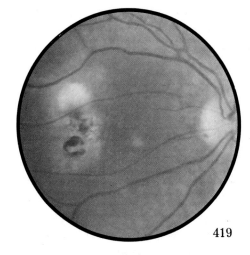

418

419

*Right eye. Central choroiditis of unknown origin, acute stage. Chorioretinal scar also present.*

*Same eye as figure 418, one month later. Choroiditis in healing stage.*

cropsia, and positive or negative scotomas, depending on the site and extension of the focal process. Pain is not present unless the condition is associated with iridocyclitis or scleritis. The inflammation may run a self-limited course, but frequently it is chronic and progressive, showing recurrent attacks. Not infrequently, however, symptomless chorioretinal scars are found on routine ophthalmoscopy.

OPHTHALMOSCOPICALLY, the choroidal lesions appear as small or large, solitary or multiple, central, peripheral or diffusely spread lesions in the fundus, all resembling each other and giving no basis for an etiological diagnosis.

In the acute exudative stage (Figs. 414, 416, 418), there is diffuse subretinal and retinal edema which is soon followed by lesions appearing as ill-defined, slightly elevated, fluffy, pale, yellowish-white patches in the fundus. In front of the patches there is usually some vitreous haze. The retinal vessels may show some perivasculitis, and the disc may be edematous.

When healing starts after some time, the fluffy patches subside and are converted into chorioretinal scars, usually seen as sharply outlined, whitish, atrophic areas with or without pigment accumulation or bordered by irregular pigment deposits (Figs. 415, 417, 419—425). The atrophic area may be avascular or crossed by fragments of the choroidal vessels.

In disseminated choroiditis the chorioretinal scars are indistinct and more or less confluent, and the pigment clumping

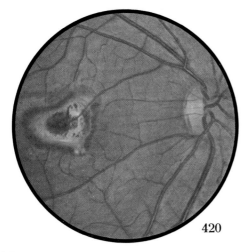

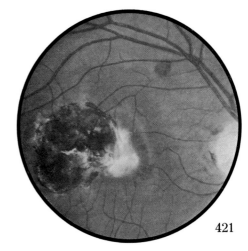

*Right eye. Central choroiditis of unknown origin, scar stage.*

*Right eye. Central choroiditis of unknown origin, scar stage.*

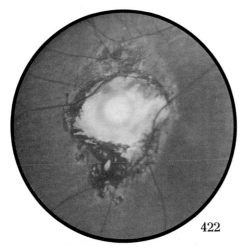

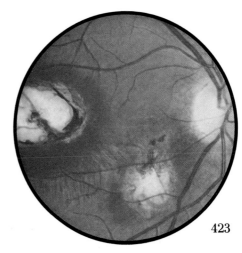

*Right eye. Circumscribed choroiditis in toxoplasmosis, scar stage.*

*Right eye. Circumscribed choroiditis in tuberculosis, scar stage.*

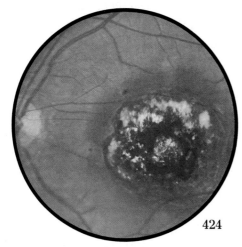

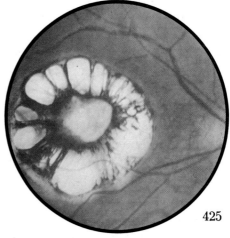

*Left eye. Old central choroiditis with massive pigmentation in toxoplasmosis.*

*Right eye. Central choroiditis in toxoplasmosis, scar stage.*

is irregular and often widespread (Figs. 426—430).

In diffuse choroiditis the fundus may assume a nearly salt-and-pepper appearance, as seen for example in intrauterine rubella infection (Figs. 431—432). The fundus may also be dotted with minute chorioretinal scars (Fig. 433) or show a more diffuse chorioretinal degeneration (Figs. 434—435) and a varying amount of pigment accumulation (Figs. 434, 436).

Occasionally, a small lesion of acute choroiditis may be confused ophthalmoscopically with a commencing malignant choroidal melanoma or a commencing disciform macular degeneration, but using fluorescein angiography it is often possible to distinguish these conditions by their different patterns of fluorescence.

In the scar stage, choroiditis should not be confused with colobomas, angioid streaks, old choroidal ruptures, fundus changes in excessive myopia or conditions associated with pigmentary degeneration in the fundus.

HISTOPATHOLOGICALLY, acute choroiditis is characterized by a granulomatous or non-granulomatous inflammation.

The granulomatous type is usually related to bacterial, viral, mycotic or parasitic inflammation, and to conditions such as tuberculosis, syphilis, toxoplasmosis, brucellosis and sarcoidosis. It consists of focal or diffuse infiltration of the choroid by epitheloid cells, lymphocytes and plasma cells. Infective agents are sometimes found in the lesion. The overlying retina usually shows considerable degeneration, and perivasculitis is found in the adjacent areas. The scar stage is

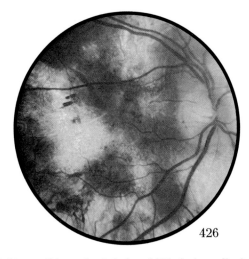

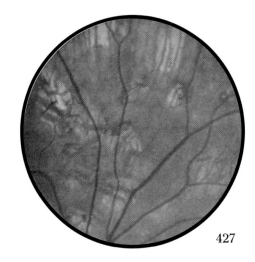

*Right eye. Disseminated choroiditis in brucellosis, scar stage.*

*Left eye. Disseminated choroiditis of unknown origin, scar stage.*

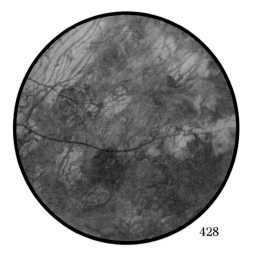

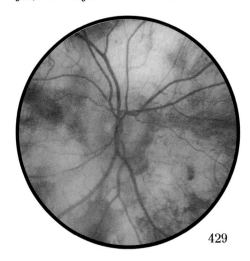

*Left eye. Disseminated choroiditis of unknown origin, scar stage.*

*Left eye. Disseminated choroiditis of unknown origin, scar stage.*

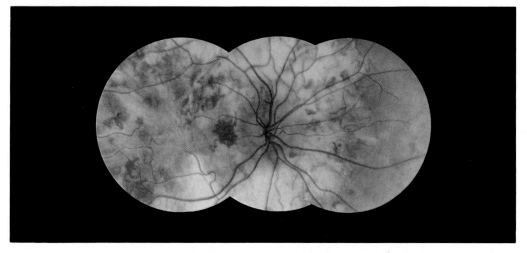

*Figure 430. Composite picture. Right eye. Disseminated choroiditis of unknown origin, scar stage. Extensive chorioretinal atrophy with pigment clumping and exposure of the whitish sclera.*

characterized by fibrosis of the choroid, destruction of retinal pigment epithelium and rods and cones, together with a varying degree of disorganization of the other retinal layers.

The non-granulomatous type is usually related to toxic or allergic insults or bacterial or viral inflammation of low virulence. It consists mainly of diffuse choroidal and retinal exudate, together with some infiltration of the choroid by lymphocytes and subsequently plasma cells. The condition subsides, leaving no or only slight degenerative changes in the choroid and the retinal pigment epithelium.

# Retinochoroiditis Juxtapapillaris (Jensen)
(Figures 437—442)

Retinochoroiditis juxtapapillaris is an inflammatory condition of unknown etiology. It is characterized by circumscribed fundal lesions, adjacent to or involving the optic disc, together with a sector-shaped scotoma, often spreading fan-wise from the blind spot, and due to a lesion of the nerve fibers. Recurrences are frequent *in loco,* but the inflammation runs a self-limited course and the visual prognosis is frequently good.

Retinochoroiditis juxtapapillaris may occur at any age, but predominantly in young adults, and is usually unilateral.

In the acute stage, there is hazy vision. Visual acuity is moderately or severely reduced and a sector-formed field defect can be demonstrated. The hazy vision disappears in the course of some weeks or a few months, and vision often becomes normal or nearly normal again unless the papillomacular bundle is damaged, but the field defect remains stationary. Recurrences are frequent *in loco* and the field defect usually remains unchanged.

OPHTHALMOSCOPICALLY, the acute stage (Figs. 437, 439, 441) is characterized by vitreous haze and diffuse edema adjacent to or surrounding the optic disc, and frequently some edema of the disc. In the edematous area there is a circumscribed

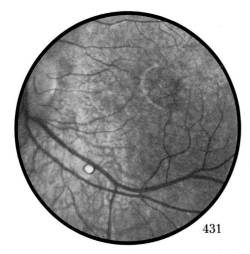

431

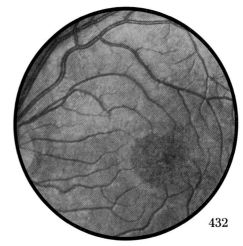

432

*Left eye. Diffuse choroiditis after maternal rubella, scar stage.*

*Left eye. Diffuse choroiditis after maternal rubella, scar stage.*

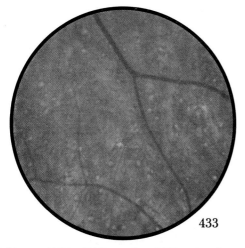

433

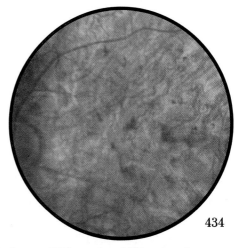

434

*Right eye (15°). Diffuse choroiditis of unknown origin, scar stage.*

*Left eye. Diffuse choroiditis of unknown origin with some pigment clumping, scar stage.*

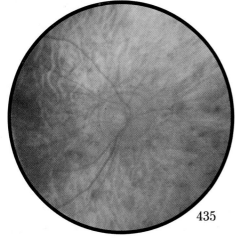

435

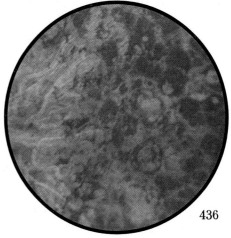

436

*Right eye. Diffuse choroiditis and optic atrophy in syphilis, scar stage.*

*Same eye as figure 435. Nasal periphery shows marked pigmentation.*

exudate of disc size or larger, often accompanied by a few retinal hemorrhages. The retinal vessels are more or less obscured by the exudate, the veins engorged and the arteries normal or slightly narrowed.

When the inflammation subsides, the exudative patch is converted into a chorioretinal scar (Figs. 438, 440—442), just as in choroiditis. In subsequent attacks (Fig. 441), new exudates appear adjacent to the chorioretinal scar.

HISTOPATHOLOGICALLY, there are too few microscopic reports to give a definitive description of the condition, but both retina, choroid and optic nerve head may be involved.

# Retinoschisis and Retinal Cysts
### (Figures 443—450)

Retinoschisis can be divided into two forms.

The juvenile or idiopathic form, which shows a hereditary tendency and often is sex-linked, affecting young males, is probably congenital in origin and due to degenerative changes both in the vitreous and the retina, resulting in splitting of the retina into two layers and the formation of cyst-like spaces which may sometimes be converted into giant cysts in the fundal periphery.

The senile form, which occurs most frequently between the ages of 50 and 70 years, is closely related to cystoid degeneration of the retina. In this condition the retina becomes split into two layers by coalescence of the cystic spaces.

Both forms are frequently bilateral and slowly progressive. The lesion starts in the fundus periphery and in the juvenile form it is often confined to the lower temporal quadrants, producing an absolute scotoma corresponding to the site of the lesion. The condition is often not noticed by the patient, and is thus first discovered on routine examination, unless the macular area is involved and central vision decreased.

Retinoschisis and a retinal cyst may be present in the same eye. The major complication in both conditions is the development of retinal detachment by the formation of holes in the outer retinal layers.

OPHTHALMOSCOPICALLY, retinoschisis is seen (Figs. 444—448) as a flat or slightly elevated area with fairly well-defined, branching whitish lines or bands lying beneath or in front of the retinal vessels, or lying as a thin opaque web (Figs. 446—447), partly obscuring the retinal vessels and protruding slightly into the vitreous. At times, the whitish lines are bordered by some pigment. In the affected area, small oval or round intraretinal cavities may be seen plainly (Fig. 443). The lesion always starts in the fundal periphery and gradually progresses towards the optic disc. In the senile form, cystoid degeneration is present in the fundal periphery.

Retinal cysts, which often occur together with retinoschisis, are most often located in the lower temporal quadrants. They appear as grayish-pink, yellowish-

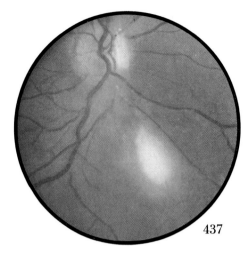

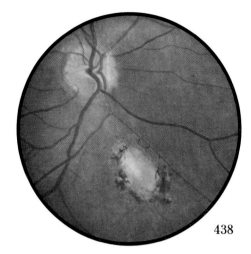

Right eye. Retinochoroiditis juxtapapillaris, acute stage.

Same eye as figure 437, four years later. Exudates converted into scars.

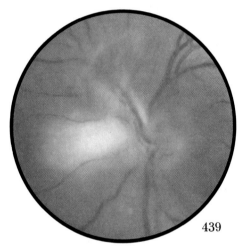

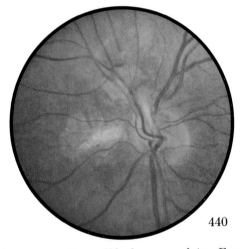

Left eye. Retinochoroiditis juxtapapillaris, acute stage.

Same eye as figure 439, three years later. Exudate converted into scar.

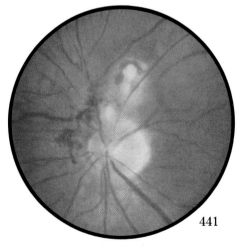

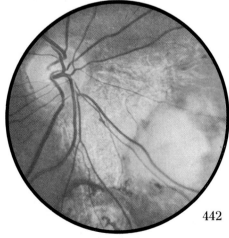

Left eye. Retinochoroiditis juxtapapillaris, acute and scar stage.

Right eye. Retinochoroiditis juxtapapillaris, scar stage.

pink or grayish (Figs. 448—450), well-defined globules, projecting forward for a variable distance and containing stretched retinal vessels in the projecting wall. At times, a tear develops in the wall of the cyst, leading to retinal detachment (Fig. 449).

In typical cases the diagnosis is not difficult. In less advanced cases, however, the diagnosis may be difficult to establish using ordinary ophthalmoscopy and is only confirmed by using the slit-lamp with a Hruby lens or the Goldmann three-mirror contact lens. In cases where retinoschisis is complicated by retinal detachment, it may be difficult to distinguish it from "primary" retinal detachment. In cases associated with retinal cysts, the condition has to be distinguished from cysts of other origin, including traumatic cysts and parasitic cysts.

HISTOPATHOLOGICALLY, juvenile retinoschisis is seen as a splitting of the retinal layers immediately under the ganglion cell layer, or even more superficially, while senile retinoschisis is seen as a splitting of the retinal layers by coalescence of numerous small cysts in the external plexiform layer, producing more or less atrophy of the other retinal layers. A retinal cyst is lined internally by a very delicate glial membrane containing the retinal vessels and externally by relatively intact neuroepithelium and pigment epithelium.

# Choroidal Detachment
## (Figures 451—453)

Choroidal detachment is a condition in which the choroid has been separated from the sclera by an effusion of fluid. It may occur spontaneously without any apparent cause, follow intraocular surgery or be related to inflammation or trauma.

Spontaneous choroidal detachment is a rare condition, most often affecting males between the ages of 30 and 60 years. The condition is frequently bilateral, and often progressive over a period of some years. Reattachment may, however, occur spontaneously after a varying number of years.

In the early stage vision is not affected, but visual field defects are present corresponding to the extension of the detachment. Later, however, central vision may be reduced or even lost.

Choroidal detachment following intraocular surgery may occur just after the operation or appear some days later, and the condition is considered among other things to be due to insufficient wound closure. The early occurrence is very common, but usually the choroid is reattached spontaneously within a few days. The choroidal detachment appearing some days after surgery occurs in about 10 to 15 per cent of the cases. The detachment usually disappears within 2 to 3 weeks.

Postoperative choroidal detachment is usually associated with diminution or abolition of the anterior chamber, lower-

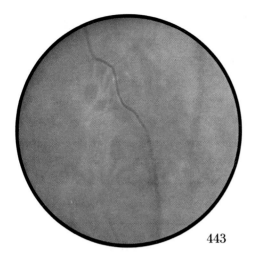

443

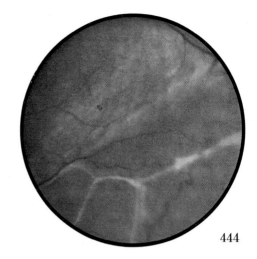

444

Right eye. Retinoschisis with network of whitish tissue and cystic spaces.

Left eye. Retinoschisis, seen as fine whitish, intraretinal lines.

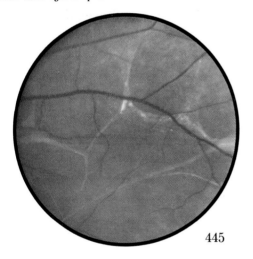

445

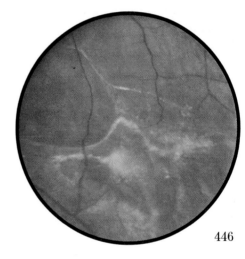

446

Figures 445 and 446. Same right eye. Retinoschisis, seen as fine, branching, whitish

intraretinal lines and diffuse whitish veils.

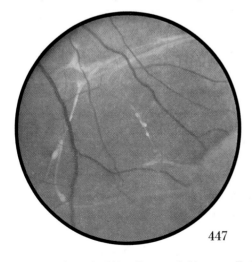

447

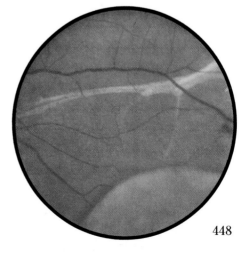

448

Figures 447 and 448. Same right eye. Retinoschisis and retinal cyst. There are several

whitish intraretinal lines, and below, there is a grayish-pink elevated area, a retinal cyst.

ing of the intraocular tension and visual field defects. If the anterior chamber remains flat for a longer period, it may result in the development of closed-angle glaucoma.

The choroidal detachment associated with inflammatory conditions or trauma is principally determined by the primary disease.

OPHTHALMOSCOPICALLY, choroidal detachment is seen as a dark grayish-brown smooth elevation in the fundus periphery or an elevation containing fine whitish parallel lines (Figs. 451—452). The lesion often shows well-defined bounderies, the convexity of which is towards the optic disc. The detachment may be confined to a single quadrant, usually the lower temporal, or may involve the whole periphery. If the detachment is extensive, the detached areas may bulge forwards like balloons separated by ridges caused by the anchorage of the vortex veins. On transillumination, the detached area usually appears lighter than the non-detached areas. The retinal vessels appear normal when passing over the detached area. On moving the eye, the lesion shows no wave-like motions as may be seen in retinal detachment. In long-standing cases clumping of pigment may occur in the affected area (Fig. 453), giving it a moth-eaten appearance.

In the differential diagnosis, retinal detachment as well as malignant choroidal melanoma have to be considered.

HISTOPATHOLOGICALLY, the choroid is detached from the sclera by an albuminous fluid and there is marked congestion and dilation of the choroidal vessels.

# Vitreous Detachment

(Figure 454)

Vitreous detachment is a common condition frequently associated with the aging process, and therefore frequently found after the age of 50 years. Vitreous detachment may, however, also occur in conditions such as myopia, and vitreous retraction may follow inflammatory or degenerative conditions.

Vitreous detachment is not infrequently associated with retinal tears, and may in some cases eventually be followed by retinal detachment.

The condition is often unnoticed by the patient, but sometimes the detaching vitreous may cause photopsia due to traction in the retina. If vitreous detachment is complicated by retinal detachment, symptoms of the latter condition will supervene.

OPHTHALMOSCOPICALLY, the condition may give rise to abnormal reflexes in the fundus, and occasionally the posterior hyaloid membrane may show some condensation (Fig. 454), seen as a slightly opaque membranous veil around the disc and the macular area, where the vitreous is firmly attached. The condition is easily recognized by using the slit-lamp together with a Hruby lens or a Goldmann three-mirror contact lens.

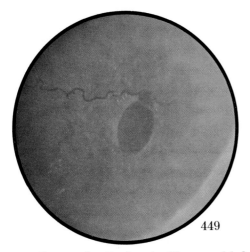

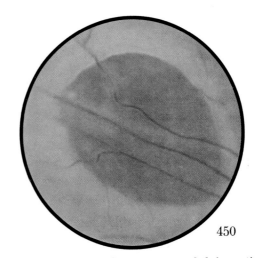

*Left eye. Ruptured retinal cyst with an oval hole.*

*Left eye. A retinal cyst surrounded by retinal detachment.*

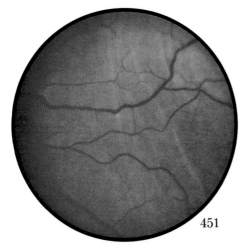

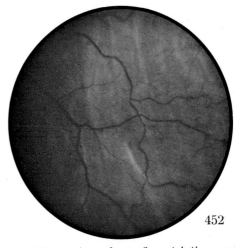

*Figures 451 and 452. Same right eye. Choroidal detachment. The detached area is slightly ele-*

*vated. The surface shows fine striation and the color is grayish-red.*

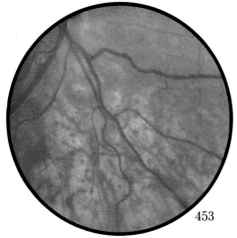

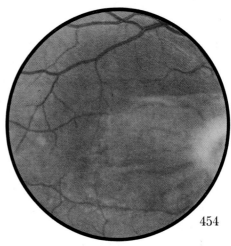

*Right eye (15°). Pigment migration in long-standing choroidal detachment.*

*Right eye. Localized vitreous detachment.*

# Detachment of the Retina
### (Figures 37—39, 148—149, 455—472 and 488)

The condition known as retinal detachment is a separation of the main retina from the retinal pigment epithelium. The separation occurs between the pigment epithelium and the layer of the rods and cones, as these layers are only loosely attached to each other except at the optic disc and the ora serrata, while the pigment epithelium is firmly attached to the choroid. The loose attachment between the pigment epithelium and the rods and cones represents a potential space, the original cavity in the embryonic optic vesicle.

Retinal detachment is probably always secondary to some local ocular disease.

In the majority of cases, detachment is due to some primary, often obscure retinal or vitreal degeneration, producing a tear or hole in the retina, through which fluid can escape into the potential space between the pigment epithelium and the neuroepithelium. This condition, often named "primary" retinal detachment, occurs most frequently in the age group between 40 and 70 years and is more common in males (60 to 70 per cent of the cases) than in females. It becomes bilateral in about 15 to 30 per cent of the cases, and is more common in myopic eyes (about two-thirds of the cases) than in emmetropic or hypermetropic eyes. Some cases show a hereditary tendency, but in most cases the hereditary element is considered to be a disposition to retinal or retino-vitreal degeneration rather than a disposition to retinal detachment itself.

In the minority of cases, in which there is usually no tear or hole in the retina, the detachment is secondary to neoplastic conditions such as retinal or choroidal tumors (Fig. 488), circulatory conditions such as angiomatosis of the retina (Figs. 148—149), toxemia of pregnancy, Eales' disease, Coats' syndrome, inflammatory conditions such as severe uveitis (Fig. 472) and sympathetic ophthalmitis. In proliferative diabetic retinopathy, Eales' disease and retrolental fibroplasia (Figs. 37—39), or following perforating traumas of the eye, retinal detachment may occur due to traction in the retina by the organized tissue. In such cases detachment is seen primarily without a retinal hole, but the continuous pull in the retina may give rise to a secondary retinal tear (Fig. 471).

Retinal detachment may also occur after ocular surgery, particularly cataract extraction. It occurs in about 2 per cent

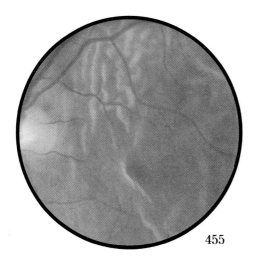

455

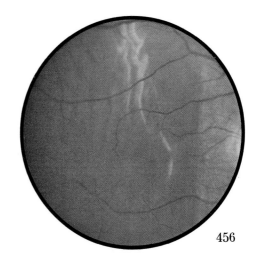

456

*Left eye. Shallow retinal detachment, recognized by wavy, whitish lines.*

*Right eye. Shallow retinal detachment, recognized by wavy, whitish lines.*

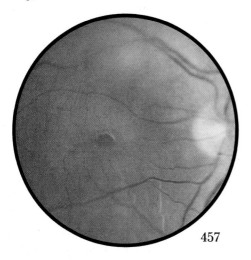

457

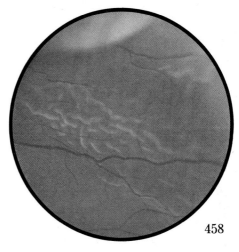

458

*Right eye. Retinal detachment with an apparent macular hole, a pseudo-hole.*

*Right eye. Retinal detachment, shallow below and prominent above.*

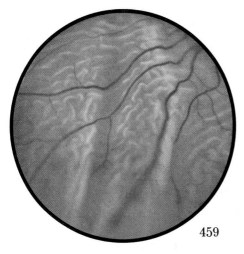

459

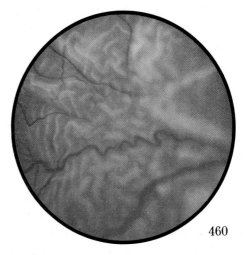

460

*Figures 459 and 460. Same left eye. Shallow retinal detachment, recognized by discrete wavy,*

*whitish lines and some bending of the retinal vessels.*

of all cataract extractions and especially in cases with loss of vitreous fluid.

A retinal detachment may appear with or without prodromal symptoms. In the former case, which is rather frequent, the patient notices some muscae volitantes, metamorphopsia and flashes or flickers of light in part of the visual field, some days or even weeks before the detachment becomes evident. The symptoms of retinal detachment may vary considerably according to the site and extension of the detachment. When detachment is large and involves the macular area, central vision becomes suddenly reduced. When detachment starts in the periphery, a cloudy shadow suddenly appears in the visual field, and as the detachment spreads towards the macula the shadow enlarges and vision becomes increasingly impaired. If, however, the detachment is flat and localized in the lower part of the fundus it may escape the notice of the patient until it is discovered on routine examination. The detachment is usually progressive, and therefore if untreated it usually becomes total and vision is lost.

OPHTHALMOSCOPICALLY, retinal detachment shows wide variations depending on the site, extension, projection and duration of the detachment, and on the site and form of the retinal tears or holes.

When a detachment has been present for some time, the detached retina loses its normal transparency and becomes visible as an opaque, grayish-white membrane. The detached area is either sharply limited, or passes without sharp limits into the attached, normal-looking retina.

In shallow or flat detachment (Figs. 455—460), the detached retina assumes a rippled surface which is recognized by discrete, wavy, whitish lines, and the retinal vessels in this area show slight bending. In deep or far projecting detachment (Figs. 461—462, 465), the retina is seen as a grayish-white, uneven membrane resembling hills and valleys, or as a large balloon sometimes obscuring the optic disc. The detached retina projects forward for a varying distance and usually shows wave-like motions when the eye is moved. In the detached area the retinal vessels appear more tortuous and darker than normal.

In the early stage, the retinal detachment is usually limited to a segment of the fundus and is often situated in the upper quadrants. As the subretinal fluid tends to gravitate to the lower part of the eye, detachment gradually becomes total. The upper part of the retinal detachment, however, often becomes flat when the subretinal fluid has settled below.

In "primary" retinal detachment, retinal tears or holes are almost invariably present (Figs. 465—470). The tears are mainly located in the equatorial region or at the ora serrata and most often they appear in the upper temporal quadrant. Frequently, more than one hole is present in the fundus.

According to size and form, the holes are classified as horseshoe-shaped tears with operculum, linear tears with serrated margins, small rounded holes occurring mainly in areas of cystoid degeneration, and arcuate holes due to disinsertion or dialysis of the retina at the ora serrata.

When the retinal tear or hole is situated in an area of far projecting detachment, it is seen plainly as a sharply outlined area through which the red color of the choroid becomes apparent, contrasting sharply with the surrounding retina. When the hole is situated in a shallow detachment or non-detached area, how-

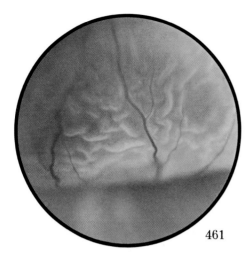

461

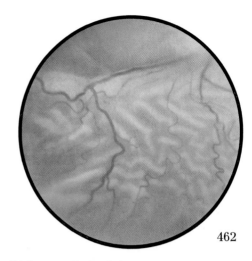

462

*Right eye. Retinal detachment, projecting forward about ten diopters.*

*Right eye. Retinal detachment. Detached retina projects about five diopters.*

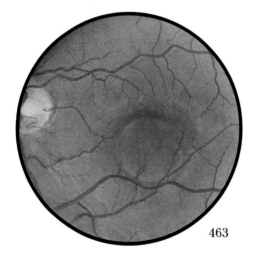

463

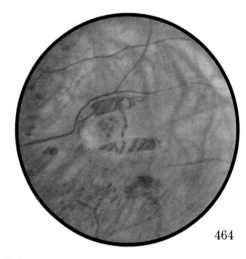

464

*Left eye. Sickle-shaped hole in the macula without retinal detachment.*

*Left eye. Horseshoe-shaped retinal tear without retinal detachment.*

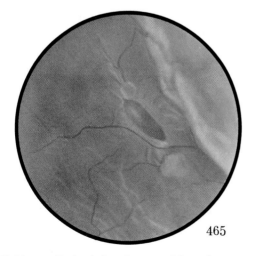

465

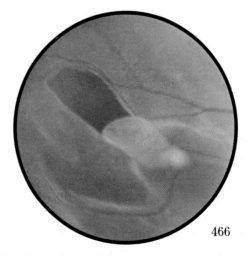

466

*Right eye. Retinal detachment with oval tear and two opercula.*

*Right eye. Retinal detachment with oval tear and whitish operculum.*

ever, it may be difficult to detect because of the small contrast in color (Figs. 463—464).

In detachment in the macular area, a distinctly outlined red patch, usually a macular pseudo-hole (Fig. 457), may be difficult to distinguish from a true macular hole.

In the diagnosis of retinal detachment, direct and indirect ophthalmoscopy and examination with the Goldmann three-mirror goniolens should always be performed to trace and localize the retinal holes very accurately as this is of greatest importance for a successful operative treatment.

In the differential diagnosis, ultrasono-graphy is of particular value because this method allows the distinction between "primary", spontaneous retinal detachment and detachment due to a solid process, usually a malignant choroidal melanoma. Transillumination as well as fluorescein angiography may also provide valuable information in such cases.

Retinoschisis and retinal cysts are discussed elsewhere.

HISTOPATHOLOGICALLY, retinal detachment is seen as a separation of the main retina from the pigment epithelium. The retinal changes are characterized by cystoid degeneration, areas of atrophy and tears. The choroid and the vitreous show various degrees of degeneration.

# Grouped Pigmentation of the Retina
### (Figures 473—474)

Grouped pigmentation of the retina is a rare congenital anomaly characterized by non-progressive patchy aggregations of the pigment in the retina. The basis of this anomaly is hyperplasia of the pigment cells of the retinal epithelium. The condition is nearly always unilateral.

The pigmentation does not cause any visual or other functional disturbances.

OPHTHALMOSCOPICALLY, the pigmentations are seen (Figs. 473—474) as sharply defined, rounded or angular, grayish-brown, dark-brown or nearly black patches, frequently grouped in a manner resembling the footprints of an animal or arranged in quite irregular masses. The size varies from small dots to disc size. The pigmentations are frequently confined to a single sector of the fundus, becoming larger as they approach the periphery. The posterior pole and the macula are usually not involved. The retinal vessels pass in front of the pigmentations.

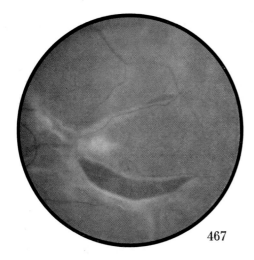

467

*Left eye. Retinal detachment with horseshoe-shaped retinal tear.*

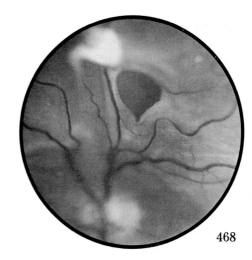

468

*Left eye. Retinal detachment and retinal tear with a whitish operculum.*

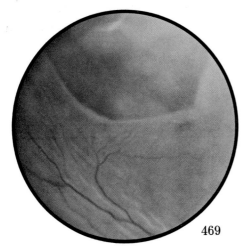

469

*Right eye. Retinal detachment with a giant tear.*

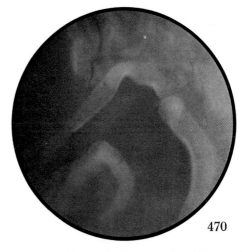

470

*Right eye. Retinal detachment with a giant horseshoe-shaped retinal tear.*

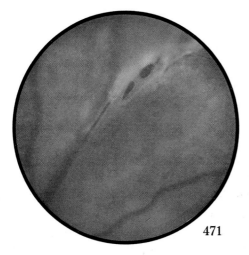

471

*Right eye. Retinal detachment with two small oval tears surrounded by connective tissue.*

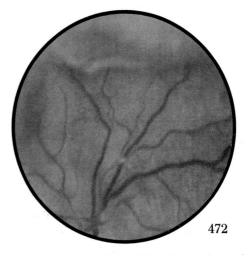

472

*Left eye. Exudative retinal detachment in uveitis.*

The ophthalmoscopic picture of grouped pigmentation of the retina is very characteristic, and should not be confused with choroidal nevi or malignant choroidal melanoma.

HISTOPATHOLOGICALLY, the condition is characterized by areas of varying size, showing proliferation and aggregation of deeply pigmented retinal pigment epithelium cells, some of which may have migrated into the retina. The overlying neuroepithelium shows failure of development of rods and cones.

# Choroidal Nevus
### (Figures 475—478)

Choroidal nevus or benign choroidal melanoma is a relatively common neoplasm consisting of melanocytes.

Choroidal nevi have a congenital basis although they do not become evident ophthalmoscopically until about puberty or during pregnancy, when all melanocytic cells of the body become active.

Choroidal nevi are usually stationary and benign, but a nevus may sometimes be transformed into a malignant choroidal melanoma.

Choroidal nevi do not cause visual disturbances. A small scotoma may, however, be present in the visual field.

OPHTHALMOSCOPICALLY, a nevus is seen (Figs. 475—478) as a flat, circular or oval, slate-gray, grayish-green or bluish patch of nearly uniform density, with ill-defined, often somewhat feathered margins and usually about the size of the optic disc. It is most frequently situated near the disc, but it may occur in the macular area or elsewhere in the fundus. The overlying retina is flat or slightly elevated, and the retinal vessels lying in front of the nevus appear darker than normal. At times, small drusen-like light dots are present on the surface of the nevus.

In the differential diagnosis of choroidal nevus, grouped pigmentation of the retina and malignant choroidal melanoma have to be considered. Ophthalmoscopically, the distinction between a choroidal nevus and a malignant choroidal melanoma is usually not difficult. In some cases, however, it may be rather difficult. In these cases fluorescein angiography may be of some help. If the choroidal lesion shows no staining it is a choroidal nevus, but if the lesion shows fluorescence the conditions cannot be distinguished by fluorescein angiography, and the patient must be kept under further control.

HISTOPATHOLOGICALLY, choroidal nevi are highly cellular tumors composed of oval or spindle-shaped, well-differentiated, mature pigment-bearing cells showing no or only few mitotic figures, and the cells do not infiltrate the surrounding tissues.

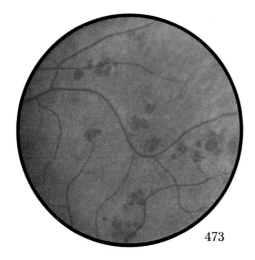

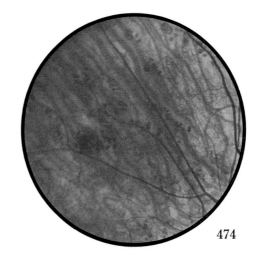

*Left eye. Grouped pigmentation of the retina like footprints of an animal.*

*Left eye. Grouped pigmentation of the retina like footprints of an animal.*

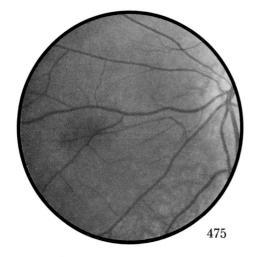

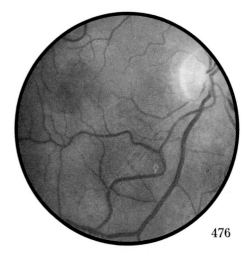

*Left eye. Choroidal nevus, seen as a flat, oval grayish-green patch.*

*Right eye. Choroidal nevus, seen as grayish-green patch of uniform density.*

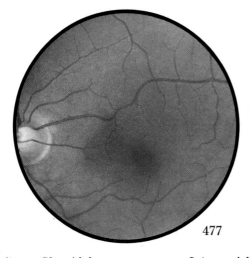

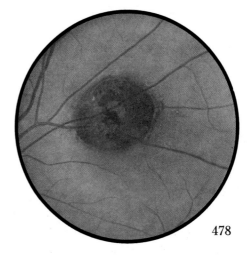

*Left eye. Choroidal nevus, seen as a flat, grayish-black area.*

*Right eye. Choroidal nevus, seen as a flat, rounded, nearly black pigmentation.*

# Malignant Melanoma of the Choroid

(Figures 479—490)

Malignant choroidal melanoma is the most common malignant intraocular neoplasm. It may arise anywhere in the uveal tract, but most often in the choroid. Bilateral occurrence is extremely rare.

The malignancy depends on the cell type. The prognosis is best in cases where the tumor is composed of spindle cells and tumors containing heavy deposits of reticulin, and poorest in mixed and epithelioid tumors, and those containing sparse or no reticulin. The average ten-year mortality rate of malignant choroidal melanoma, including all cell types, is about 50 per cent.

Malignant melanoma occurs most frequently in middle life, and is exceedingly rare in children.

The symptoms depend on the site and extension of the tumor. Tumors localized at or near the macula early give rise to metamorphopsia, blurred vision and central scotoma. Tumors localized elsewhere in the fundus may be unnoticed for a long time, but sooner or later give rise to defects in the visual field. Secondary glaucoma may sometimes develop as a result of intraocular extension of the tumor. Occasionally, the tumor causes an intraocular hemorrhage with a sudden loss of vision.

Extraocular extension of the tumor and metastases may occur early, and may occasionally be the first sign of a malignant choroidal melanoma. The tumor extends along the ciliary nerves and vessels, or infiltrates the sclera directly. Invasion through the substance of the optic nerve into the meninges is unusual. The metastases are hematogenous. They may involve almost any organ of the body, but most frequently the liver.

OPHTHALMOSCOPICALLY, malignant melanoma is seen in the early stage as an indistinctly outlined, often mottled, yellowish-red, grayish or brownish, flat or slightly elevated patch in the fundus, and the retinal vessels overlying the tumor appear darker than normal (Figs. 479—480). As the tumor grows, extension takes place in the plane of the choroid (Figs. 481—484) and towards the retina (Figs. 486—487). When the tumor has penetrated Bruch's membrane, the retina is pushed forwards (Figs. 488—489) and detached to a variable extent, but retinal tears or holes are usually not present. The color of the tumor varies with the degree of pigmentation, from yellow or yellowish-pink to grayish-red or even dark brown, but the color is usually not uniform, as the pigment is irregularly distributed.

In malignant choroidal melanomas penetrating into the vitreous, pigmented tumor cell aggregations may occasionally be dispersed into the vitreous or diffusely spread on the retinal surface (Fig. 485).

A benign medulloepithelioma, which is a rare condition, may ophthalmoscopically be indistinguishable from a malignant choroidal melanoma (Fig. 490).

Malignant choroidal melanoma can be both easy and difficult to diagnose. In early stages, it may be confused with a

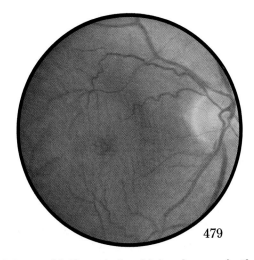

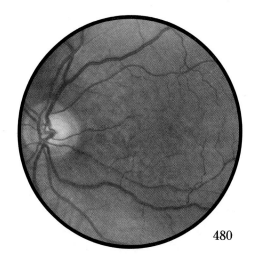

479

480

*Right eye. Malignant choroidal melanoma in the macular area.*

*Left eye. Malignant choroidal melanoma seen as flat grayish-green tumor.*

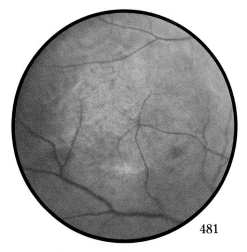

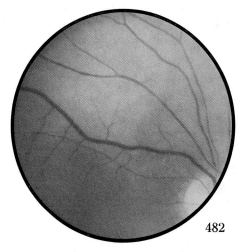

481

482

*Right eye. Malignant choroidal melanoma seen as flat yellowish-gray tumor.*

*Right eye. Malignant choroidal melanoma seen as yellowish-green tumor.*

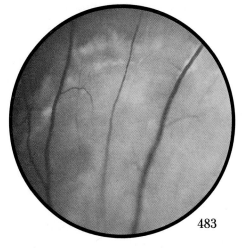

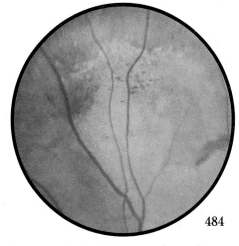

483

484

*Right eye. Malignant choroidal melanoma seen as flat yellowish tumor.*

*Right eye. Malignant choroidal melanoma seen as flat yellowish tumor.*

choroidal nevus, commencing disciform degeneration of the macula, subretinal hemorrhage, metastatic carcinoma of the choroid, angioma of the choroid, acute choroiditis or tuberculoma of the choroid. In the late stages, it may be confused with simple retinal detachment, detachment of the choroid or cysts of the retina. Complicating secondary glaucoma, intraocular hemorrhage, uveitis or panophthalmitis may also make the diagnosis difficult. A blind and phthisic eye should always arouse suspicion of malignant choroidal melanoma.

In the diagnosis of malignant choroidal melanoma, direct as well as indirect ophthalmoscopy should be performed together with transillumination of the eye and slit-lamp examination aided by a Hruby lens or a Goldmann three-mirror goniolens.

Fluorescein angiography may be of value in the diagnosis and differential diagnosis, as some of the conditions to be considered often show characteristic patterns of fluorescence different from those in malignant choroidal melanoma (commencing disciform macular degeneration, acute choroiditis, and, sometimes, choroidal angioma), or show no fluorescence (subretinal hemorrhage and, frequently, choroidal nevus).

Using ultrasonography it is possible to distinguish between a solid process and simple retinal detachment.

Finally, the color and growth of the patological process is of great value in differentiating the conditions.

Melanin in the urine is probably only present when extensive metastases are present.

HISTOPATHOLOGICALLY, malignant melanomas are classified according to the cell type as spindle A and B, fascicular, mixed and epithelioid tumors. The tumors are usually highly cellular, containing varying amounts of reticulin and often showing areas of necrosis.

## Metastatic Carcinoma of the Choroid
(Figures 491—492)

Metastatic tumors in the choroid may arise from carcinoma, hypernephroma, malignant melanoma or chorionepithelioma. Although rare, metastatic carcinoma is the most common secondary tumor in the choroid.

Metastatic carcinomas of the choroid are the results of emboli of malignant cells reaching the eye through the posterior ciliary vessels. Lodged in the choriocapillaris, the cells multiply and infiltrate the choroid, forming a secondary tumor.

The most frequent site of the primary carcinoma is the breast and the lung. However, the primary tumor may also be a carcinoma of the gastro-intestinal tract, kidney, prostate, ovary, parotid gland, liver, testicle, pancreas or thyroid.

The occurrence of visual disturbances depends exclusively on the site and extension of the choroidal metastases. There may be no ocular symptoms, or a history of failing vision in one eye. Bilateral occurrence, however, is not infrequent. Symptoms of secondary glaucoma and

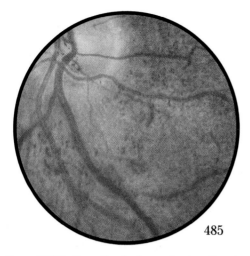

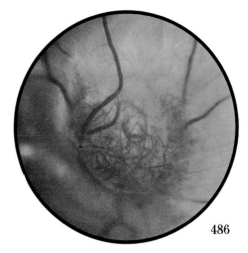

485

*Left eye (15°). Preretinal pigment migration from malignant melanoma.*

486

*Right eye. Malignant choroidal melanoma obscures the optic disc.*

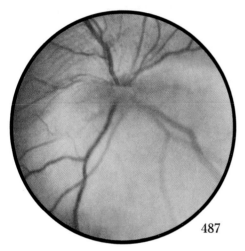

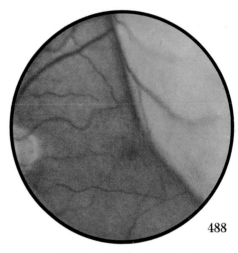

487

*Right eye. Malignant choroidal melanoma seen as prominent mass below.*

488

*Left eye. Malignant choroidal melanoma and some retinal detachment.*

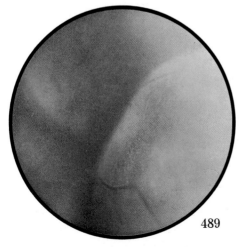

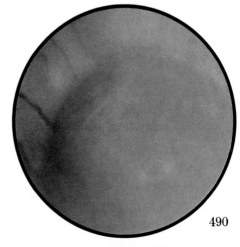

489

*Left eye. Malignant choroidal melanoma seen as a prominent mass.*

490

*Left eye. Benign medulloepithelioma seen as a large, prominent mass.*

pain sometimes become evident in the late stages, but these symptoms may occur earlier if the ciliary body and iris are affected.

OPHTHALMOSCOPICALLY, metastatic choroidal tumors are seen (Figs. 491—492) as well- or ill-defined, rounded, slightly raised, opaque, often mottled, grayish, yellowish or yellowish-white areas of varying extension. They are either single or multiple, and typically they appear on the temporal side near the optic disc. Small hemorrhages may occur but they are not a prominent feature. The metastases extend chiefly in the plane of the choroid with relatively little increase in thickness. Sometimes, a shallow, more or less wide-spread retinal detachment may develop.

In typical cases presenting a history of carcinoma elsewhere, the diagnosis is not difficult. In cases with no apparent primary tumor, however, the condition has to be differentiated from malignant choroidal melanoma, acute choroiditis and the acute stage of retinal arterial occlusion.

HISTOPATHOLOGICALLY, the cells of a metastatic carcinoma of the choroid are often less differentiated than those of the primary tumor. It may be difficult or impossible, therefore, to determine the site of the primary carcinoma by examining the metastatic tumor.

# Fundus Changes in Retrobulbar Tumor
### (Figures 493—494)

Any orbital tumor of sufficient size may cause indentation of the eye and give rise to retinal folding or ridging.

OPHTHALMOSCOPICALLY, the indentation is seen in the fundus as horizontal or slightly oblique, parallel retinal folds or ripples (Figs. 493—494), most often situated in the macular area. When the tumor is removed the folds usually disappear, unless permanent shrinkage has developed.

# Retinoblastoma
### (Figures 495—499)

Retinoblastoma is a retinal tumor composed of undifferentiated neuroblastic cells, and occurring most frequently in childhood. The tumor is probably always congenital in origin, and bilateral in about 20 to 25 per cent of the cases. In bilateral cases, the extension of the tumor is often different in the two eyes when noticed, or the tumor may be unilateral at first observation, and not appear in the second eye until months or even years after the tumor is noticed in the first eye. Although most cases are sporadic, familial cases occur. The off-

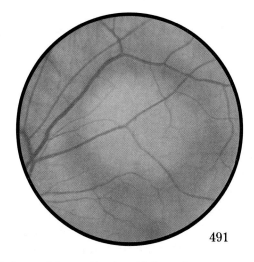

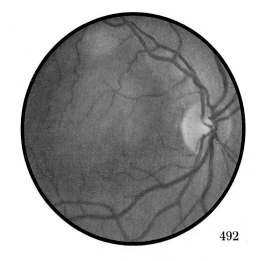

491

492

*Left eye. Metastatic choroidal carcinoma, seen as rounded, yellowish area.*

*Right eye. Metastatic choroidal carcinoma seen as yellowish areas in the macula.*

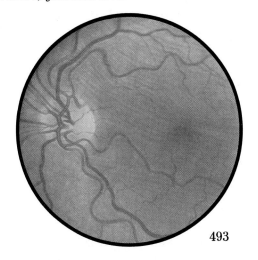

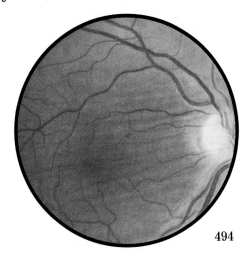

493

494

*Left eye. Retinal ridging from an orbital tumor.*

*Right eye. Retinal ridging from an orbital tumor.*

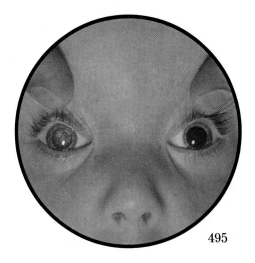

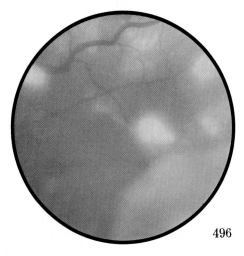

495

496

*Retinoblastoma, seen as an yellowish-pink mass through the right pupil.*

*Left eye. Retinoblastoma. Several ill-defined, whitish retinal tumors.*

spring of survivors of the disease show a rather high incidence of retinoblastoma.

Most frequently, retinoblastoma is observed clinically during the first four years of life. After that age, the incidence declines abruptly, and it is extremely rare in adults.

As retinoblastoma occurs predominantly in small children, the first evidence of disease is frequently observed by the parents as lack of fixation, development of strabismus and most frequently as an anomalous whitish pupillary reflex, known as "amaurotic cat's eye" (Fig. 495).

The tumor may spread within the eye by local extension producing an enlargement of the globe, an endophthalmitic reaction in the eye or even painful secondary glaucoma. Most frequently, the tumor spreads by direct extension along the optic nerve, reaching the intracranial cavity. Less frequently, it penetrates the walls of the bulb into the orbit and the surrounding structures. In these cases lymphatic spread may occur along the orbital lymphatics, at first to the preauricular and cervical lymph nodes and later showing a more diffuse involvement of the lymph nodes. Hematogenous metastases are common and involve primarily the bones and the viscera, especially the liver.

The prognosis after careful treatment of the tumor in the early stage is fairly good, but in advanced cases with extension into the orbit, into the central nervous system, or where metastases have appeared, the condition is invariably fatal in spite of any treatment.

In successfully treated cases of retinoblastoma, the patient should be examined at short intervals for a period of at least two to four years, as new tumor growth may occur in the treated eye or in the previously unaffected eye.

OPHTHALMOSCOPICALLY, a retinoblastoma is seen in the early stage as a sharply defined, rounded, yellowish-white, grayish-white or pinkish-white tumor of varying size, situated anywhere in the fundus. The irregularly projecting surface of the tumor shows fine tortuous vessels (Fig. 498), often also pearly-white, calcareous deposits and, occasionally, small hemorrhages. The tumor may be single (Figs. 497—498) or present a number of lesions of similar size, or consist of a larger lesion surrounded by several small ones (Fig. 496).

The tumor growth may be either endophytic or exophytic.

In the former case, tumor growth takes place on the anterior surface of the retina, proliferates into the vitreous, and tumor implants may be seeded anywhere in the unaffected parts of the retina. Occasionally, a vitreous haze due to an endophthalmitic tumor reaction may partly obscure the fundus.

In the latter case, tumor growth takes place on the posterior surface of the retina and is therefore not as easily detected as the endophytic type of extension. In the early stages, exophytic extension appears as an elevated grayish zone in the fundus. In the later stages it is accompanied by a progressive detachment of the retina.

When the tumor has grown sufficiently large it becomes visible to the naked eye as a whitish pupillary reflex, the well-known condition of "amaurotic cat's eye" (Fig. 495).

After successful treatment, the retinoblastoma subsides, leaving an atrophic zone and often some calcareous deposits (Fig. 499).

In the diagnosis, scleral transillumination, ultrasonography and sometimes

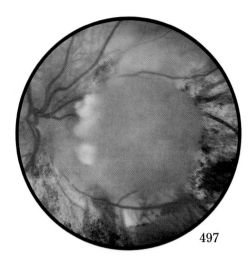

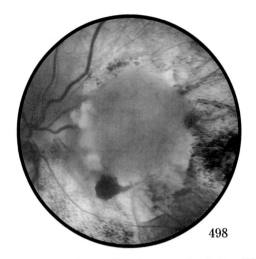

497

498

*Right eye. Retinoblastoma, seen as a prominent grayish-red tumor.*

*Same eye as figure 497, four months later. The tumor is in regression.*

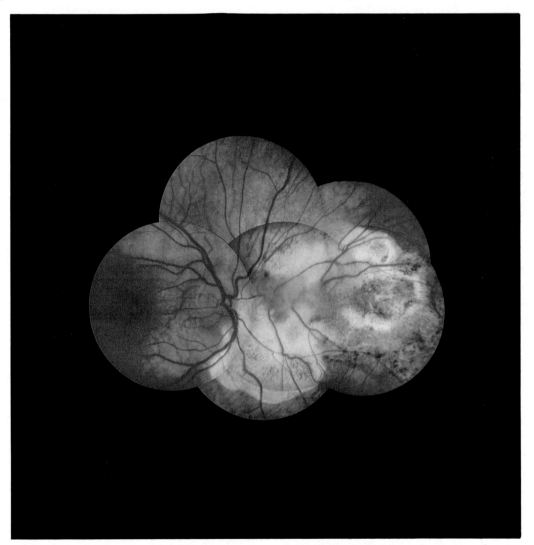

*Figure 499. Composite picture. Same eye as figure 498, four months later. The tumor has completely disappeared and there is a large area of chorioretinal atrophy.*

fluorescein angiography may be of value.

The early diagnosis of retinoblastoma is of great importance. The diagnosis may sometimes, however, be difficult and the condition may be confused with non-malignant conditions such as Coats' syndrome, angiomatosis of the retina, choroidal tuberculoma, persistence of the primary vitreous, retrolental fibroplasia, falciform retinal detachment and endophthalmitis.

HISTOPATHOLOGICALLY, a retinoblastoma is composed principally of undifferentiated neuroblastic cells which exhibit large hyperchromatic nuclei and scanty cytoplasm. The tumor cells show a varying degree of differentiation and have a tendency to form retinoblastoma-rosettes. There are usually numerous mitotic figures, and areas of necrosis are often present, except in the perivascular area.

# Mechanical Injuries to the Eye
## (Figures 500—519)

Mechanical injuries to the eye are common. They may involve every structure in the eye and be the result of contusion and concussion or due to perforating or penetrating lesions.

In the anterior part of the eye, the most common lesion due to contusion is anterior chamber hemorrhage (hyphema), rupture of the root of the iris (iridodialysis), rupture of the sphincter of the iris and luxation of the lens. Perforating wounds most often result in prolapse of the iris and in cataract.

In the posterior part of the eye, contusions may result in retinal edema, macular cyst- or hole-formation, retinal or choroidal hemorrhages, and choroidal ruptures. Perforating lesions following accidents or foreign bodies cause hemorrhage and varying degrees of tissue damage. Retinal detachment may be a late complication.

Traumatic retinal edema, also known as commotio retinae or Berlin's edema, is the most frequent retinal lesion resulting from blunt injury. Usually it develops within 24 hours after the injury and disappears in the course of some days or weeks. While the edema persists, visual acuity is reduced and field defects are present. When the edema subsides, normal vision is often restored.

OPHTHALMOSCOPICALLY, traumatic retinal edema is seen (Figs. 500—501) as a grayish-white or grayish, opaque, ill-de-

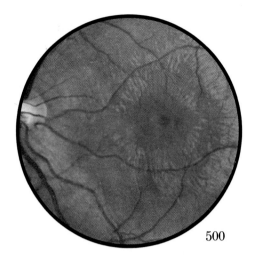

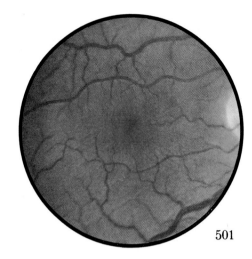

500

501

*Left eye. Traumatic macular edema seen as a grayish, ill-defined area.*

*Right eye. Traumatic macular edema, in subsidence.*

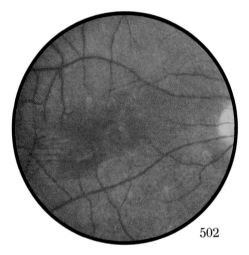

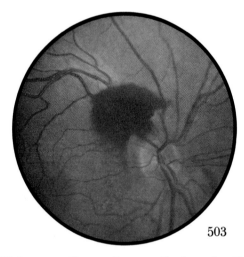

502

503

*Right eye. Traumatic macular pigmentation and depigmentation.*

*Right eye. Traumatic preretinal and retinal hemorrhages.*

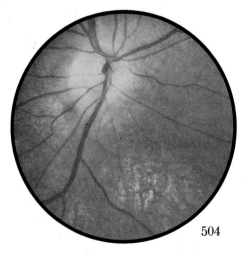

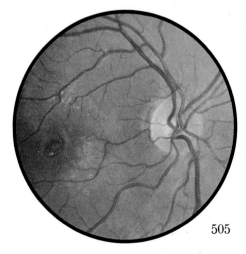

504

505

*Right eye. Atrophic fundal areas after traumatic retinal hemorrhage.*

*Right eye. Traumatic macular hole surrounded by slight retinal folding.*

fined, slightly elevated area most often situated in the posterior part of the fundus. The fovea is likely to appear as a cherry-red spot and the macular area is often surrounded by linear light reflexes (Figs. 500—501). The edema usually disappears leaving no trace, but sometimes the edema may result in permanent degenerative changes, including pigmentary abnormalities (Fig. 502) or macular cyst- or hole-formation (Fig. 505), with permanent impairment of central vision.

Retinal or preretinal hemorrhages (Fig. 503) may also be the result of a blunt injury. These hemorrhages often subside leaving no trace, but pigmentary changes (Fig. 504) may occasionally follow the hemorrhage.

Traumatic choroidal ruptures are frequently obscured in the acute stage by intraocular hemorrhage. The ruptures are first discovered when the vitreous clears in the course of some days or weeks.

OPHTHALMOSCOPICALLY, traumatic choroidal ruptures are seen (Figs. 506—507, 510—511) as crescentic or irregular white patches or lines of exposed sclera, commonly situated within 3 or 4 mm from the disc. Usually there is only a single choroidal rupture (Fig. 510), but several ruptures may be present in the same fundus (Figs. 507, 511). The ruptures are most frequently seen at the temporal side of the disc and not infrequently they may involve the macular area (Fig. 511). In the early stage, the rupture is surrounded and partly obscured by retinal and subretinal hemorrhages and by retinal edema (Figs. 508—509). In the scarring stage, the lesion is seen as an elongated, usually crescentic, whitish or grayish-white atrophic zone with a varying amount of pigment deposits (Figs. 510—511).

Intraocular foreign bodies (Figs. 512—513) may cause more or less extensive damage to the structures of the eye. Pigmentary changes and scar formation may

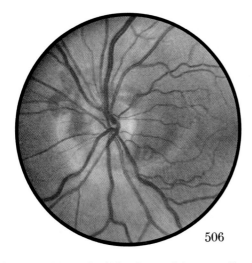

506

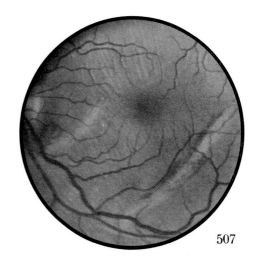

507

*Figures 506 and 507. Same left eye. Fresh choroidal ruptures, seen as a whitish crescent* surrounding the lower part of the disc and a whitish line outside the macula.

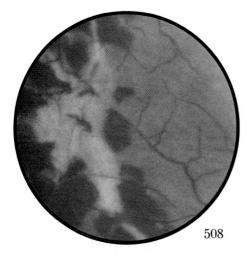

508

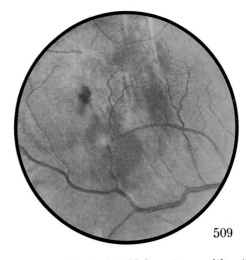

509

*Right eye. Fresh choroidal rupture partly obscured by hemorrhage.*

*Right eye. Fresh choroidal ruptures with retinal edema and hemorrhage.*

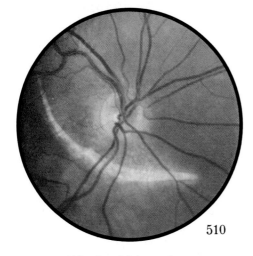

510

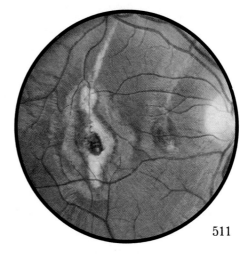

511

*Right eye. Old choroidal rupture, seen as a whitish crescent.*

*Right eye. Old choroidal ruptures with some pigmentation in the macula.*

occur after the foreign body has been removed (Figs. 514—515).

Retained intraocular foreign bodies of iron often cause siderosis, while retained foreign bodies of copper may cause diffuse intraocular degeneration (chalcosis) or a violent uveitis with subsequent phthisis. In early stages of siderosis, the electroretinogram is of the negative plus type. Later, it changes to the negative minus type, and finally the electroretinographic response becomes extinguished. If the foreign body is removed in the first stage, the electroretinogram may be normalized.

Perforating lesions (Figs. 517—518) may result in gross intraocular hemorrhage and more or less extensive damage to the structures of the eye, followed by scar formation (Fig. 519), and later in some cases by retinal detachment.

In rare instances, the perforating lesion may give rise to the occurrence of papilledema ex vacuo (Fig. 516).

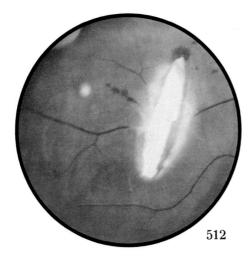

512

*Left eye. Metallic foreign body in the fundus.*

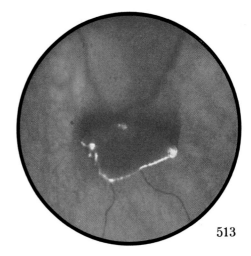

513

*Left eye. Metallic foreing body lying preretinally, partly obscured by hemorrhage.*

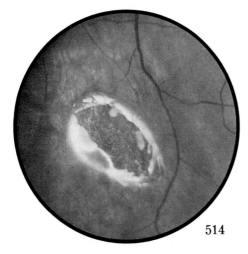

514

*Right eye. Remnants of fibrin cap, which had obscured metallic foreign body.*

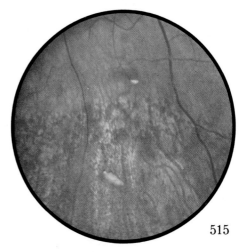

515

*Same eye as figure 514, a fortnight later. The fibrin has been absorbed.*

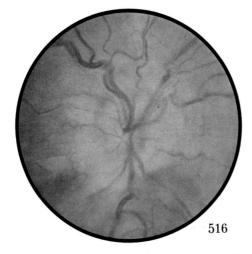

516

*Right eye. Papilledema ex vacuo. Optic disc swollen and veins engorged.*

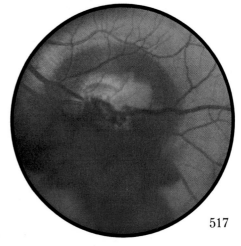

517

*Left eye. Perforating lesion with subretinal and preretinal hemorrhage.*

# Purtscher's Retinopathy
### (Figure 520)

Purtscher's retinopathy, angiopathia retinae traumatica or retinopathy due to distant injury, is a condition occurring in association with injury to the skull or thoracic compression. The nature of the condition is not quite clear and, therefore, still a matter of discussion.

The condition appears within a few days after the injury and usually subsides within a few weeks.

In the acute stage, visual disturbances may occur if the macula is involved, but these disturbances usually disappear when the retinopathy subsides.

OPHTHALMOSCOPICALLY, the condition (Fig. 520) is characterized by woolly exudates and streaky hemorrhages, usually within the area bordered by the superior and inferior temporal vessels. The hemorrhages and exudates gradually become absorbed, usually leaving no trace.

# Fundus Changes after Strangulation
### (Figure 521)

Fundus changes after strangulation are seldom observed, but may occur in the form of small or large retinal, preretinal or subretinal hemorrhages (Fig. 521).

# Sun Eclipse Injury of the Retina
### (Figures 522—523)

Every sun eclipse is watched by many people. In spite of warnings, some people do not wear dark, protecting lenses and some may afterwards show retinal lesions following the thermal effect of the sun.

Visual disturbances due to this thermal effect may occur as central scotomas or scotomas elsewhere in the visual field.

OPHTHALMOSCOPICALLY, the condition is seen in the scarring stage (Figs. 522—523) as a chorioretinal lesion with atrophy and pigment accumulations, preferentially in the macular area.

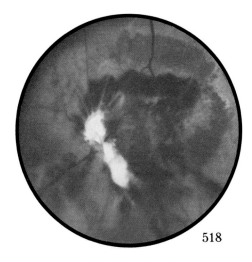

518

*Right eye. Perforating fundus lesion partly obscured by hemorrhages.*

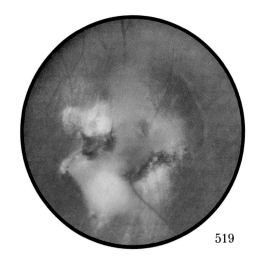

519

*Same eye as figure 518, four years later. Atrophic scar and vitreous opacities.*

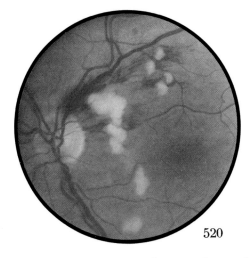

520

*Left eye. Cotton-wool exudates and streaky hemorrhages in Purtscher's retinopathy.*

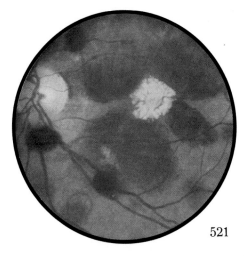

521

*Left eye. Preretinal, retinal and subretinal hemorrhages after strangulation.*

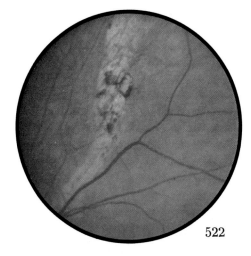

522

*Left eye. Sun eclipse injury, seen as an elongated chorioretinal scar.*

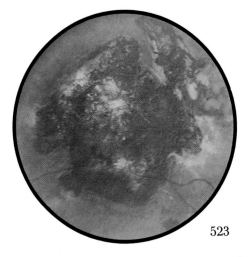

523

*Right eye. Sun eclipse injury, seen as a large macular chorioretinal scar.*

# INDEX

Numbers without parentheses refer to figure
numbers.
Numbers in parentheses refer to page numbers.